Medicinal and Aromatic Plants

Medicinal and Aromatic Plants

O.P. Thakur

AMIGA PRESS. INC
Delhi -110051

AMIGA PRESS. INC
H.O :- 28-A, Indra Park, Chander Nagar
Delhi :- 110051 (India)
Tel :- 011-22504028, +91-98736-57000
Email :- amigapress@gmail.com
Website :- www.amigapress@co.in

This edition is published by Amiga Press.Inc

ISBN : 978-93-84533-12-0

First Published 2018

PRINTED : REPLIKA PRESS PVT. LTD.

Preface

Medicinal plants are nature's hidden and to a large extent unexplored treasure. Although they have been used as a source of safe and effective medicine since time immemorial, this potential resource has hardly been commercially tapped. India is endowed with about 8000 species of medicinal plants. According to a recent estimate of the Planning Commission, Government of India, the potential for plant-based crude drugs is about Rs. 400 billion. Globally, the demand for medicinal plants and their derivatives is growing at a rate of 7-15%.

The medicinal properties of plant species have made an outstanding contribution in the origin and evolution of many traditional herbal therapies. These traditional knowledge systems have started to disappear with the passage of time due to scarcity of written documents and relatively low income in these traditions.

Over the past few years, however, the medicinal plants have regained a wide recognition due to an escalating faith in herbal medicine in view of its lesser side effects compared to allopathic medicine in addition the necessity of meeting the requirements of medicine for an increasing human population. Through the realization of the continuous erosion of traditional knowledge of plants used for medicine in the past and the renewed interest at the present time, a need existed to review this valuable knowledge of medicinal plants with the purpose of developing medicinal plants sectors across the different states in India. Our major objectives therefore were to explore the potential in medicinal plants resources, to understand the challenges and opportunities with the medicinal plants sector, and also to suggest recommendations based upon the present state of knowledge for the establishment and smooth functioning of the medicinal plants sector along with improving the living standards of the underprivileged communities.

The aromatic plants possess odoriferous and volatile substances which occur as essential oils, gum exudate, balsam and oleoresin in one or more parts, viz. root, wood, bark, foliage, flower and fruit. The chemical nature of these aromatic substances may be due to a variety of complex the chemical compounds. Many of these aromatics are powerful germicides and have anti-bacterial properties, but the bulk of the produce finds use in perfumery and the food-flavouring industries. Amongst the two, the per fumeru and allied industries consume much larger amounts of the natural fragrant material. According to the UN Word Statistics

(1972), the annual world trade (excluding countries in eastern Europe) in essential oils and perfummery aromatics for 1969 was of the order of Rs 2250 million; also, a large quantity of the aromatic material of plant origin is utilized in cosmetics, toiletries and allied industries. Our current volume of foreign trade in the perfumery material, essential oils and aromatic compounds is around Rs 65 million and this amount accounts for 1. 6 per cent of the world trade. Some sixty-two types of essential oils come to the international market with a large and consistent demand. However, our treatment of the aromatic plants is confined to a few more important essential-oil crops grown in the country.

The methods employed to obtain aromatic substances from plants are classified into distillation, enfleurage, maceration, expression and solvent extraction. Expect in the case of flowers crops, such as jasmine and kewara in which the fragrant constituents are likely to be decomposed or destroyed, the essential oils are mostly obtained by distilling the produce; in fact, steam distillation is the oldest method of separation of essential oils. The perfumery material is filled in a large-galvanizediron still over a perforated netal grid. Water is filled in the still below the level of the grid so that it generates a low-pressure steam on heating to pass through the material. The water vapours carry with it the essential oil of the perfumery material. These vapours are passed through a condenser and collected in a vessel where the oil is ecanted with a separating-funnel.

This book may be able to provide a lucid discourse on the subject to the person seeking a brief information on the topics.

—Editor

Contents

1

Medicinal Properties of Astavarga Plants

Various Ayurvedic Nighantu books composed or commented by different Vaidyas over several centuries describe the medicinal properties of all the Astavarga plants either as a group or alone are reproduced hereunder. Till date none has tried their chemical evaluation in the modern laboratories. Certainly, as is evident, they need further investigation on scientific lines to add value to their excellent text described qualities. The Astavarga plants have been described under three Ayurvedic terms that is Jeevniya, Brhneeya, Vayaasthapan. It is therefore essential to explain them before proceeding to give their medicinal properties.

Jeevaniya are those plant drugs which strengthen the bodily Vitality (Prana Shakti) through their action on three humours (three doshas —vata, Pitta, Kapha) bringing them into equilibrium state — described in Ayurveda as a state of perfect health.. Plants described as Jeevaniya, in various Nighantus are Jeevak, Rishbhak, Meda, Mahameda, Kakoli, Kshirkakoli, Mugdaparni, Mashaparni, Jeevanti and Yastimadhu. These medicines also enchance anabolic activities over the catabolism in the body.

Brhneeya **:**The drugs which promote the formation of mansa dhatu that is flesh formation. Such drug plants are ksirini, Dugdhika, Aswagandha, Kakoli, Kshirkakoli, Sweta Bala, Peet Bala, Van Kapas, Vidari, Vidhara.

Vaya Sthapan (Gerontologic) **:**These plant drugs clears the body of three doshas and particularly the Vata dosha and thus does not allow progressive growth changes to occur or if they occur it is at a very slow rate. This means that the immunity system becomes strong and metabolic processes are growth promoting. The plant drugs in this category are Meda, Mahameda, Rdhi, Vrdhi, Amalaka, Guruchi, Punarnava, Shatavari, Jeevanti, Haritaki, Sweta Aprajita, Mandukaparni and Shalparni.

Jeevaka **:**is sweet (madhur), refrigerant, pacifies pitta, Rakta and vata doshas. It is useful in burning sensation, fever and consumption, increases kapha dosha and sukra (seminal fluid) (Gana Nighantu). Nighantu Ratnakar states that it is madhur, sheetal, shukrajanak, kaphakarak, Rakta pitta nashak, Balkarak (tonic) and is useful in treating vata, pitta, fever (jvar), Krsta (emanciation), phthisis, burning sansation and blood disorders.

Rshbhak is sweet in taste and pacifies pitta, vata and rakta doshas. It is useful in consumption, burning sensation in the body, fever and increases kapha dosha and Shukradhatu (Nighantu Ratnakar).

Both Jeevak and Rishbhak are nutritious, tonic, refrigerant, viryavardhaka, madhur and are useful in pitta dosha, burning, blood disorder, vata dosha and consumption (Bhava Prakash).

Meda **:**In Nighantu Churamani it is stated that meda is sweet, sheetvirya, it pacifies pitta dosha, increases kapha and shukra. It is useful in phthisis, burning sensation in the body and fever. Nighantu Rantnakar describes its properties as sweet in taste, sheetal, guru, dhatuvardhaka, increases milk in ladies, Snigdha, kaphakarak and is useful in vata, pitta, rakta vikar, consumption, fever, burning sensation in body and cough.

Mahameda is madhur in taste, sheetal, increases kapha and shukra. It pacifies pitta dosha, and is useful in burning sensation of the body, blood disorders, consumption and fever due to vata dosha (Dhanwantri Nighantu, Raj Nighantu). Both Meda and Mahameda increases meda dhatu in the body.

Rdhi is paustik, tridoshnashak, Shukrajanak, madhur, guru, vitality enhancing prana (Pranaprada). Aishwarya janak and is useful in epilepsy, rakta —pitta doshas —(Bhava Prakash). In Nighantu Ratnakar it is written that it is sweet in taste, unctous, medha janak, sheetal, kaphakarak, sukravardhaka, pranadayaka, Balkarak, Rakta shodhak, Ruchikarka, guru and is useful in leprosy, worm infestation, epilepsy, raktapitta thirst, consumption, pitta, vata, rakta dosha and fever.

Vrdhi is cooling nutritious, causing conception, Shukra vardhaka, pacifies rakta pitta doshas, ulcers in stomach, cough and consumption ("Shaligram Nighantu ").

Kakoli **:**The roots are sweet in taste, slightly bitter, refrigerant, galactagogue, fatty and is useful in phthisis, pitta, pains due to vata aggravation, blood problems, burning sensation in the body and fever. It increases kapha and shukra dhatu. (Dhanwantri Nighantu). It is vata —pittahar, Sheetal, Brhna and cures emaciation due to consumption (Madan Pal Nighantu). In Nighantu Ratnakar, it is mentioned that it is Sheetal, Vrsya, madhura, tikta, kaphakari, guru, destroys phthisis, pitta, thirst and is beneficial in rakta dosha, raktapitta, emaciation, visam jwar, and aggravated vata-pitta.

Kshirkakoli **:**The bulbs are sweet slightly bitter, refrigerant, expectorant, antipyretic, aphrodisiac, galactagogue and tonic. It is useful in cough, general debility, fever, vitiated condition of pitta, seminal weakness, burning sensation, increases vitality (Madan Vinod Nighantu, Sodhal Nighantu, Raj Nighantu, Kaidev Nighantu, Dhanwantri Nighantu).

Astavarga is cooling, tasty, nutritious tonic, aphrodisiac, nourishes body and increases kapha. It is beneficial in seminal weakness, increases fat in the body, heals bone fracture and cures vata, pitta, and rakta doshas, abnormal thirst, burning sensation in the body, consumption, fever and diabetic condition. It is one of the excellent combination of herbal drugs which restores health immediately, strengthens immunity system and rectifies defects in anabolism or body growth processes and works as antioxidant in the body. That is why Aswani Kumars invented it for curing the frail, emaciated sick body of Chayavan Rishi who regained youthful condition it is claimed. There is need to grow these species on large scale to take up clinical trials and chemical investigations. The tissue culture programme may be advantageous to save these species and achieve fast multiplication.

Botanical Description with Characters of Drug Part of Astavarga Plants

Vrdhi – (Habenaria acuminata Lindl. syn.

Habenaria edgeworthii Hook. f. ex Collett) :

Stem – 30 to 60 cm.. high. leafy, stout

Leaves – Ovate, oblong-lanceolate, 4-10 cm long acute, acuminate thick, upper leaves gradually smaller, nerves 5-7, base sheathing.

Flowering Spike – 7cm to 25cm long,, bearing many flowers.

Flowers – Yellow green 1 to 1. 5cm across with lanceolate acute bracts, the lower shorter, the upper longer, than the ovary sepals green, pubescent, the margins slightly fringed; petals yellow thick, erect; lip yellow, longer than the sepals concave narrowing to a long strap shaped limb; Spur about twice the length of ovary, yellowish –green curving upwards with tip curved down.

Flowering & Fruiting time – July –August.

Characteristics of usable drug part – Tubers are in pair the older becomes Shrivelled as the growing period proceeds. The shape of the tuber is oval to ovate and slightly tapering at the opposite end giving it a shape resembling to cotton boll. Skin dull white, flesh white and sweetish-bitter in taste.

Distribution

Himachal – Summer Hills,, Shimla; Mountains near Manali, Rahla Forest, Kothi, Manali, Sarahan, Nirmand-Annu, Rwanda, Kamarunag peak, Saptasar above Rawalsar (Mandi), Chansel, Churdhar, Jangtoo, Chamba, Narkanda.

Uttaranchal-Mussoorie-Jaberkhet, Mussoorie, Kyarphulli, Company Bagh, Deoban, Tehri-Nagtibba West of Dhanolti; Uttarkashi-Jamuna Valley, Kharshali,

Har-Ki-Dun; Chamoli-Valley of flowers, Gobindghat, Khirsu; Pithoragarh-Tejam Jankhola Vally, Kali Valley, Sarju Valley, Nainital-Nainital, Bhowali, Ramgarh, Fatehgarh, Above Malli Tal; Almora-Binsar, Almora, Lorakhet, Ranikhet to Chaubatia.

Ayurvedic drug properties :– It is emollient, aphrodisiac, rejuvenating and tonic and is beneficial in aggravated vata and pitta, burning sensation in the body, hyperdipsia, fever, cough, epilepsy, insanity, emanciation and general debility (Bhav Prakash, kai, Nirs, so, Ni, Ni, Ra)

Substitutes-Varahi Kand ((Tacca aspera Roxb.) salam panja (Dactylorhiza hatagirea) Mahabala (Sida acuta, seeds of Sida cordifolia).

Status-It is a rare species because grows in assocaiton with grasses and is being cut in early stages before seeds are mature.

Rdhi –(Habenaria intermedia D. Don)

Stem-Erect, 25-60cm high, terete, robust, leafy.

Leaves-Scattered usually 5-nerved, ovate-lanceolate acuminate, cordate at the base.

Raceme-2-6 flowered.

Flowers-5cm across white or greenish-white few, distant. Bracts leaf like lanceolate, acuminate, equal or more than ovary. Sepals persistent, 20-25mm long, green, spreading tips reflexed, upper one white inside. Petals white, 5-nerved. Lip 3-lobed, longer than sepals, green spur 5-6cm stout, longer than ovary more or less curved. Side lobes deeply fringed. Flowering time-July-August Characteristics Usable Drug Part-Tubers are round at the opposite end but tapering towards stem joint. Skin is dirty white, flesh white and is slightly bitter in taste.

Distribution-Himanchal Pradesh, Koti (Shimla) Summer Hill Indian Institute of Advance study, Kamana Hill), Rwanda and Kamarunag (Karsog), Rewalsar hills (Mandi), Shimla (Fagu), Dalhousie (Chamba), Kinnaur.

Jammu &Kashmir-Azmabad, Poonch, Pirpanjal Range.

Uttaranchal-Dehradun-Mussoorie (Jaberkhet), Camel back road, company bagh, Bhatta Fall, Kampty fall; Tehri (Nagtibba) Suakholi, Chamoli-on way to Kedarnath, Jangal chatti, way to valley of flowers, Gaurikund (Rambera); Utarrkashi-Tons Valley, Bhagirathi valley and way to Dodital.

Ayurvedic Medicinal Properties

Rdhi is Sheetvirya, pacifies vata, pitta, rakta doshas. It is useful in consumption and fevers. It increases kapha dosha and shukra dhatu. It is intellect promoting, aphrodisiac, rejuvenating, tonic and cures emaciation, epilepsy, cough, skin diseases, haematemesis and general debility.

Substitutes :-Varahi Kand (Tacca aspera Roxb.) Utangan seeds (Blepharis edulis Pers.) Bala (Sida cordifolia), Chiriya Musali (Asparagus filicinus Buch. -Ham.)

Jeevak —(Malaxis acuminata D. Don)

Syn. Microstylis wallichii Lindl.

Stem-5 to 25 cm, ribbed bearing pseudo bulbs

Leaves – Usually 3 may be more,, 5-10cm ovate-lanceolate, acute with prominent veins and light green.

Flowers – Shortly stalked about 10mm in diameter, yellowish-green with purple centre. Sepals oblong, 2 lateral rather shorter than the dorsal, margins recurved. Petals linear longer than sepals, margin recurved. Lip shied-like, slightly convex, tip notched or bilobulate, auricles straight and slightly over lapping.

Flowering Time-July-August.

Characteristics of Usable Drug Part

Pseudo bulbs are in pair and new formation looks like a garlic clove (hence called rasona kand vat). Colour is green white and these remain alive over long period. Flesh is bitterish in taste.

Distribution:-Himalaya, Khasihills (Meghalaya) Andaman Islands, Travencore, Mdhya Pradesh. In Himalaya 1850 m to 2300 m Himachal Pradesh to Arunachal Pradesh, Assam, Nagaland, Manipur, Mizoram, Tripura.

Himachal Pradesh:-Shimla-Glen, Boileaugunj, Elysium Hill in forests, way to Rani forest, way from Khajiar to Chmba, Chail, Hattoo, Narkanda.

Uttaranchal :-Dehradun-Camel back road, Below Mussoorie bypass road, above barlowgunj, chakrata, Jaunsar, Tehri (Magra); Pauri-Pode khal, Chamoli-Nagnath; Ukhimath, Gopeshwar, Pithoragarh-Sarju Valley, Berenag, Thal Kedar; Nainital, Bhowali, Ramagarh, Almora-Ranikhet, Between Ranikhet-Chaubatia.

Ayurvedic Medicinal Properties :-It is sheet virya and calms down vata, rakta and pitta doshas and is beneficial in burning sensation of the body, fever, and consumption. It increases kapha and Shukra dhatu. It is aphrodisiac and tonic. It cures haematemesis, aggravated vata and pitta doshas, seminal weakness, dipsia, emaciation, tuberculosis and general body weakness. It increases body flesh and is jeevniya.

Substitutes :-Vidari kand, Bahaman Safed (Centaurea behen Linn.), Guruchi (Tinospora cordifolia)

Rshbhak-(Malaxis muscifera (Lindl.)

Kuntze- Synonym Microstylis muscifera Lindl.

Stem – 3 to 25cm high with ovoid pseudo bulbs

Leaves-One or two (unequal) 3-10 x 2-4cm sessile, ovate to ovate-lanceolate obtuse, narrowed at base to sheathing petiole.

Inflorescence-10 to 25 cm. long.

Flowers :3-4 mm long, pale-yellow-green, Bracts lanceolate shorter than ovary sepals broadly lanceolate. Petals linear Shorter than sepals. Lip ovate abruptly pointed, margins thickened.

Flowering Time-July –August.

Characteristics of the usable drug Part-Tubers round, shining white bearing stem giving shape of bullock horn having a similar curvature. The taste is slightly bitter with mucilaginous substance.

Distribution-Himalaya between 1800-3500m eastward to Sikkim.

Himachal Pradesh-Shimla (Mashobra, Fagu, Hattoo forests) Rahala forest, Dhanchoo, Sangla, chamba.

Jammu &Kashmir-Gulmarg, Datni, Leh.

Uttaranchal-Pithoragarh-Tejum Haya, Bakariudiyar, Ralam Valley, Palangarh, Ralam, Almora-Dwali, Dehradun-Chakrata, Deoban Tehri-Masartal, Bokhills, Dhanolti, way to Nagtibba; Chamoli-Vasukital, Bajmora, Jumma Area, Dunagiri, Valley of flowers, Rambara, Hemkund; Uttarkashi-Jamuna Valley above village kharsil.

Ayurvedic Medicinal Properties-Tubers are efficacious cure for pitta, rakta, vata doshas. It is useful in phthisis, burning sensation in the body, fever and increases Kapha and shukra. It is styptic, aphrodisiac and tonic. It is an effective cure in vitiated pitta and vata, seminal weakness, dysentery, emaciation and general debility.

Substitutes:-Vidari Kanda (Pueraria tuberosa DC.) Bahaman Lal (Centaurium roxburghii (G. Don) Druce), Vansalochan.

Status:-Malaxis muscifera is also a rare species and at present its reasons are not clear.

Kakoli —(Roscoea alpina Royle, Roscoea procera Wall.)

Stem-6-20cm and 30-60cm, robust.

Leaves-2-6 lanceolate, 15x3 cm.

Flowers-Several lilak, purple or white, corolla tube much longer than the calyx, borne in a short stem with or without leaves, upper lobe (petal) rounded, hooded and narrower reflexed lateral petals. Lower staminode 5x3cm obscurly 3-lobed spreading, notched at the tip.

Flowering Time-July –August or June for R. alpina.

Characteristics of the usable drug part-Fingers replacing roots are thickened 3-4 and have sickle shape, white and flesh inside is also white, tastes sweet resembling shatavar.

Distribution-Western Himalaya 1000 to 2700m commonly found in these altitudes in Himachal Pradesh, Jammu and Uttaranchal (Joshi Math, Mussoorie) and in other all districts.

Ayurvedic Medicinal Properties-Root fingers are sweet sheetvirya, pacifies vata pitta, fever due to vitiated vata-pitta. It is beneficial in consumption, burning sensation in body, increases Kapha dosa and shukra. It is also an effective cure for pains due to pitta, vata, rakta dosha, thirst due to pitta, rakta pitta etc.

Substitutes-Aswagandha (Withania somnifera) Curculigo orchioides (Kali musali)

Kshirkakoli —(Lilium polyphyllum D. Don)

Stem-30 to 100cm high, erect.

Leaves-Sessile, alternate or nearly opposite or whorled, narrow lanceolate or linear 7cm-13cmx 5mm-12mm. Bracts leaf like whorled.

Flowers-Solitary, racemed or whorled stalked (3cm-10cm), Perianth 6cm-8cm long, green-white with purple dots inside. Stigma 3-lobed, capsule 2cm to 3cm.

Flowering Time-15June-15 July

Characteristics of Usable Drug Part-The bulb is a loose mass of fleshy scales white in colour and is sweetish bitter in taste.

Distribution-Himachal-Hattoo peak, Narkanda forests, Chail (Solan district), Sungari-Bahli on Rampur Road.

Jammu & Kashmir-Gulmarg, Liddar Valley.

Uttaranchal-Gangotri, Rainthal, Amardhar, Kedarnath, Madmaheshwar. It is a rare species and its populations are very small that is 10-15 plants.

Ayurvedic Medicinal Properties- It promotes appetite and pacifies vata, pitta, rakta dosas. It is efficacious in bleeding disorders, cardiac diseases, dyspnoea, cough, consumption and diseases of urine system and is vrsya (tonic). Bulbs are refrigerant, galactagogue, expectorant and aphrodisiac. They are useful in bronchitis, burning sensation, hyperdipsia, rheumatalgia and general weakness in the body.

Substitutes- Aswagandha (Withania somnifera Dunal), swet musali (Chlorophytum arundinaceum), Fritillaria roylei Hook. f., Fritillaria oxypetala Royle.

Comments on Lilum Polyphyllum Don-Sir Col. Henry Collett (1902) wrote Flora Simlensis and in frontispiece he gave a diagram of this plant species and also mentioned under the description of species in family Orchidaceae that it is common in Shimla woods. But a search of this plant species in forests in and around was futile because even a single plant specimen was not found. This is because of disturbance in natural habitat and changing ecological conditions. Similar experience was felt in some other habitats in Uttaranchal especially in Ponwali Kanta, Rainthal area. The species has become rare and need immediate action for its conservation.

Meda —(Polygonatum verticillatum Allioni)

Stem-30cm to 1. 20m, erect, angled, grooved and sometimes mottled.

Leaves-in whorls of 4-8 sessile, linear, 10-20cm long and 5-13mm broad or lanceolate 8cm x 18mm, tips usually acute, sometimes obtuse or slightly enrolled to the midrib.

Raceme-whorled 2-3 flowered.

Parianth-5mm white often greenish

Berry-6-7mm in diameter green and red or orange on ripening.

Flowering &Fruiting Time-July-September

Characteristics of the Usable Drug Part- Plants bear rhizomes as under ground part which resemble ginger but comparatively much less thick except in very old (7-8 years) plants. The rhizomes are white or dull white in colour but flesh inside is white and is sweet in taste when dried.

Distribution- The species is widely distributed in temperate Himalaya between 1600m and 3500m.

Himachal Pradesh – Shimla,, Narkanda, Hattoo, Churdhar, Janjelli, Sikari Tibba, Kamarunagh.

Jammu & Kashmir- Trikuta Hills, Udhampur, Doda area.

Uttaranchal- Ponwalikanta, Tali, Amardhar, Ganganani dhar, Rainthal, Kedarnath, Gangotri, Madmaheshwar.

Ayurvedic Medicinal Properties- Meda rhizomes are sweet in taste sheetvirya, pacify pitta dosh and increase kapha and shukra dhatu. They are beneficial in phthisis, burning sensation in the body, and fever (Dhan. Ni.). They are emollient, aphrodisiac, tonic, galactagogue, and beneficial in aggravation of pitta, cough, ulcers, skin diseases, general debility and vulnerary.

Substitutes- Asparagus racemosus Dunal (Shatavari), Salam misri (Eulophia campestris Wall).

Mahameda —(Polygonatum cirrifolium Royle)

Stem- 30 to 130cm tall, terete, round or grooved, climbing by means of tendril like tips of the leaves and grow generally in association with bushes. leaves-are always in whorls of 3-6, sessile, linear, 5cm to 8cm long and 3-5mm broad, lower surface glaucus, the margins usually inrolled to the midrib.

Racemes- Whorled 2-4 flowered.

Parianth- 5mm white often greenish or slightly purple.

Berry- 6-7mm in diameter, green and on ripening Orange-Red.

Flowering & Fruiting Time –July-September

Characteristics of the usable Drug Part- The rhizomes generally look like ginger but less thick, white or dull white in colour and are sweet in taste on drying.

Distribution- Temperate Himalaya 1500m to 2700m

Himachal Pradesh- Shimla, Matiana, Narkanda.

Uttaranchal- Mussoorie, Chakrata, Gaurikund, Rambara, Harshal, Ganganani, Devban, Rainthal, Mandakini Ghati, Bhilangana Ghati, Ponwali, Kalimath.

Ayurvedic Medicinal Properties- According to Dhanwantri Nighantu, Mahameda is sweet in taste, sheet virya, increases Kapha and shukra dhatu and is beneficial in consumption burning sensation, and fever. Various Nighantus describe its properties as emollient aphrodisiac, galactagoue, tonic and useful invitiation of vata-pitta, strangury seminal weakness, anorexia and general body weakness.

Substitutes- Shatavari (Asparagus racemosus Willd.) Nagbala (S. Veronicaefolia Linn.) Shakaakul mishri (Polygonatum multiflorum (Linn.) All.), Paederia foetida Linn. (Prasarani).

Status- It is also a rare species because of early cutting before Seeds are mature and burning of grassy plots for removal of bushes.

Henbane: Qualities and Benefits

Family name: Solanaceae. black colored henbane Latin name: Hyoscyamus Niger Linn

Sanskrit: Prasik Yamani, Madakarani, Turushka

Hindi: Khurasani Ajwain

Gujarati: Khurasani Ajmo

Marathi: Khuasani Oba

Bengali: Khurasani Yamani

Telangi: Khurasani Vamu

Dravidi: Kurishani Vanam

Arabian: Teralbanj, Bajul

French: Tukhme Bunj, Bunj

Punjabi: Khurasani Ajwain

The plants of Henbane are found in the Garhwal regions of northern India and grow up to a height of 800 to 10, 000 feet. They are cultivated in Saharanpur, Kolkata, Agra, Ajmer, Pune and government parks and fields.

Chemical Composition

The seeds have 25 to 30 per cent oil; the leaves and flowers have hiosimine and alkaline called hiosan along with atopin and scopin in little quantities. The biannual atropine plants grow in mud.

External Form

The plants are longer than the plants of thymol seeds, annual or biannual. The roots have fibres and round in shape, straight and strong. The leaves are broad and long, with sharp edges, green in colour. The branches also have fibres. The flowers grow in bunches in yellowish colors with violet stripes. The fruits are small, there are two segments at a distance of half inch and each section has black coloured henbane with flat shape.

Qualities

1. It is dry, bitter and pungent, hot. It has alcoholic affect and causes anxiety. It cures kapha, respiratory problems, heart pain and sexual problems.
2. It is curative hence beneficial in case of piles, pain in the stomach early ejaculation, dreams, menses. painful discharge of menses and irregular menstrual cycle. It calms down the sexual desire as well.
3. Henbane has alcoholic tendency and causes urination. If taken in small doses it reduces the pace of heart beat at night and strengthens but excess quantity is harmful for the heart.
4. The weariness effect is seen on the brain, genital organs and intestines. Opium and thorn apple are similar medicines but opium causes constipation, whereas henbane is free from this quality. Thorn apple leads to drowsiness and illusions but this herb does not have any such effect hence henbane is considered to be a betzer medicine. It is the best medicine for sleepiness and getting rid off weariness.
5. It has an effect on the nervous system. It calms down the mind, gives good sleep.

Medicinal Use

Toothache: Grind henbane with leaves and keep it on the cavity to get rid off toothache.

Joint pain: Boil it in sesame oil. Massage the painful area to cure joint pain. sciatica pain and backache etc.

Ear pain: Boil henbane in sesame oil and our feu drops in the ear to cure ear pain.

Liver pain: Lep with this oil cures chronic liver er pain and chest pain.

Bleeding gums: Rinsing the mouth With the kwath (decoction) of henbane leaves stops bleeding from the gums.

Urinary Problems: The extract of henbane seeds is beneficial in case of stones, pain or burning sensation. It causes urination and thereby reduces the pain.

Anxiety:-Add 30 drops of henbane juice in 25ml of water and should be administered to patients at an interval of one hour. This is very effective in case of hysteria, lunacy and other vata related doshas.

Worms: The male having worms in the stomach should eat jaggery on empty stomach and then take henbane churna with stale water. The worms present in the intestines will come out through stools.

Uterus pain: Make a long stick with the henbane powder and insert it in the vagina.

Stomachache: Make a pill with jaggery and henbane and take to control stomachache. Alternatively add black salt in henbane churna and take it.

Add one gram dry ginger powder in two to four drops of henbane oil and eat it and drink hot aniseed extract over it, this controls stomachache immediately or add little amount of jaggery in its kwath and take it.

Cough, hiccups and vomiting

1. Keep henbane and sugar candy in a betel leaf and suck the juice to cure dry cough caused due to vata.
2. Keep the henbane seeds in mouth and suck the juice to stop hiccups caused after meals.
3. Grind the top portion of henbane and clove and lick with honey to cure vomiting.

Dysentery: Take equal quantities of henbane, ginger, tea and mochrasa, make a fine powder. Take 2 to 3 grams with water less curd, it stops dysentery.

Stones: Take 5 gm of henbane churna with 20 gm of radish juice to dissolve stones.

Worms: Grind the henbane or give its fumigation in the rectum of children to get rid off small white worms.

Leprosy: Take henbane churna with jaggery for seven days and maintain strict diet.

Piles: Make a poultice of henbane and give fomentation on the piles and with salt it calms down the urinary pain.

Fever due to indigestion: Swallow four henbane seeds with cold water without chewing it. It can also be taken with honey.

Wounds: Grind it with little jaggery and tie a poultice with rapeseed oil to heal the wounds quickly.

MEDICINAL PLANTS

- Conservation of natural resources and the capability to utilize them in sustained manner are essential for the well being and continued survival of man.
- Under the duress of over exploration and habitat degradation a number of wild plants are essentially facing a constant threat of extinction.

- Out of the 60, 000 plant species that are listed as threatened of extinction, over 20, 000 (or more) are from India alone.
- The botanical survey of India has prepared a provisional list of threatened plants which includes a large number wild (or) wild relatives of food, horticultural, medicinal and aromatic plants.
- India is endowed with a unique wealth of biota which inlcude a large number of medicinal and aromatic plants.
- Many of these plants are rare and endemic and found only in wild sources.
- The population explosion coupled with the improved standard of living led to ruthless exploitation, resulting in the imminent danger of extinction of these plants.
- Most of these wild medicinal and aromatic plants are highly habitual specific, found only in forests and occupying highly specialized ecological niche with restricted distribution.
- There are neither biological informations nor adequate knowledge of casual factors that led to their rarity in the habital.
- There is however, now an urgent need to evolve a sound strategy for the management and conservation of these plants on a long term basis.
- To evolve suitable strategies for conservation (or) the domestication/ cultivation of medicinal plants, it is very essential to study the complete biological and ecological back ground of these species.
- Under domestication outside their normal ecological range (or) under the distributed eco-system conditions may of the wild medicinal and aromatic plants tend to behave differently.
- In some cases it becomes difficult to grow them (or) it may not even survive.
- In certain other cases if survives and grows but may not be producing the desired traits.
- A through understanding on their reproductive and growth biology as well as identification of the biological and ecological constraints leading to their reduced fitness, restricted distribution (or) even extinction etc., is therefore, necessary.
- An understanding of the biological and ecological back ground of the species in their normal habitat is also essential to understand their conservation biology as well as to predict their behaviour under artificial cultivation.

Strategies for conservation of medicinal plants:

- The conservation of the wild medicinal plants or any other such threatened species can be tackled by scientific techniques as well as social actions.

- There are basically two scientific techniques of conservation of genetic diversity of these plants.
- They are the in situ and ex situ method of conservation.

In Situ conservation:

- It is only in nature that plant diversity at the genetic, species and ecosystem level can be conserved on long-term basis.
- Unless plant populations are conserved in the wild, that is in natural habitats, in viable breeding populations, they run the risk of extinction.
- It is necessary to conserve in distinct, representative biogeographic zones inter and intraspecific genetic variation.

Current status:

- In Karnataka, Kerala and Tamil nadu and more recently in Maharashtra the forest department in collaboration with FRUHT (Foundation for Rural Revitalization of Local Health Tradition) have established a network of 33 "Medicinal Plants Conservation Areas" (MPCAs) across the entire altitudinal range of south India.
- Each of these reserves is around 200 ha in size.

Regulation and wild collection:

- Regulating the harvest of medicinal plants from the wild for commercial purposes.
- Particularly those species whose harvest inevitably involves destructive collection.
- Local communities can develop a stake in sustainable harvesting of medicinal plants from the forest and village, district and state level co operative are set up to manage collection, storage and marketing.

Current status:

- LAMP societies as they function at present neither benefit the primary tribal collectors nor provides adequate powers (or) accountability of the LAMPs with regard to protection and management of forests.
- The marketing function of LAMPs is also weak, so that collectors do not get remunerative prices through LAMP sales.

EX situ conservation

A. Ethno-medicinal plant gardens:

- Creation of a network of regional and sub-regional ethno-medicinal plant gardens which should contain accessions of all the medicinal plants known to the various ethnic communities in different regions of India.
- This chain of gardens will act as regional repositories of our cultural and ethno-medicinal history and embody the living traditions of our socity's knowledge of medicinal plants.

Current status:

- There are estimated to be around 50 such gardens in the country ranging from acre to 40 acres some of them were set up by an All India Health Network.
- More recently a network of 15 such gardens have been set up in 3 states of South India with the initiative of FRLHT. One of the gardens is located in TBGRI, (Tropical botanical garden research institute) Palode at Thiruvananthapuram.

B. Gene banks:

- While it is known that the largest proportion of local bio-diversity in all our eco-system is used for medicinal purposes, very little is known about their conservation status in the wild.
- What is likely is that a large number of medicinal plant species are under various degrees of threat.
- The precautionary principles would suggest that an immediate and country-wide exercise be taken up to deposit seeds of wild medicinal plants with a first priority to known Red listed species and endemic species.

Current status:

- The department of bio-technology, Government of India has recently taken the initiative to establish 3 gene banks in the country.
- One is with ICAR at the NBPGR (National Bureau of plant genetic Resources) Campus, the second is with CIMAPs, (Cental Institute of Medicinal and Aromatic plants) Lucknow and the third with TBFRI in Thiruvananthapuram.

C. Nursery network:

- The most urgent and primary task in order to ensure immediate availability of plants and planting materials to various user groups is to promote a nation wide network of medicinal plant nurseries, which will multiply all the regional specific plants that are used in the current practice of traditional medicine.

Current status:

- Planting material for 40 odd species of medicinal and aromatic plants is reportedly available in the ICAR and CSIR (CIMAP) network.
- In South India FRLHT has recently set up a network of 55 supply nurseries.

D. Cultivation:

- Figures projecting demand and trade in medicinal plant species globally indicate a step upward trend in the near future.
- One estimate puts the figure of world trade in medicinal plants and

related products at US $ 5 trillion by A. D. 2050 (world bank report, 1996).

- The demand so far has been met mainly from wild sources.
- This can't go on for much longer; policy intervention is urgently needed to encourage and facilitate investments into commercial cultivation of medicinal plants.
- Cultivation of medicinal plants however, is inversely linked to prevalence of easy and cheap collection from the wild, lack of regulation in trade, cornering of the profits from wild collection by a vast network of traders and middlemen and absence of industry's interest in providing buy-back guarantees to growers.

Current status:

- In the Govt. sector agro-technology of 40 odd species has been developed by ICAR-Agricultural University System and CSIR (CIMAOs & RRL, Jammu and Jorhat).
- In recent years industries like Dabur, Zandu, Indian Herbs, Arya Vaidya Shala, and Arya Vaidya Pharmacy and others have made some symbolic efforts to initiate cultivation.
- Since 1984 NABARD (National Bank of Agricultural and Rural Development) has formulated schemes for financing cultivation and processing of medicinal plants.

E. Community based enterprises:

- The income generated by the traditional medicine industry benefits small section of the socity.
- A strong case exists for promotion of community level enterprises for value addition to medicinal plants through simple, on site techniques like drying, cleaning, crushing, powdering, grading, packaging etc.
- This will also increase the stake of rural communities in conservation and change the skewed nature of income distribution of the industry.

Current status:

- Three community based enterprises are known in south India, one in Gandhigram Trust, (Dindigul), Preemade development Society (Peermade) Kerala and the third by VGKK in B. R. Hills, Mysore.

MEDICINAL PLANTS IN SOUTH INDIA

In India about 7300 plant species are used in traditional health care systems such as Ayurveda, Siddha, Unani and folk healing practices. The booming of traditional medicine industry results in an increasing demand on medicinal plant products. 90% of the medicinal plants come from natural habitats. The declining availability of such plants and the fading of local traditional knowledge make the sustainable management of natural habitats a crucial environmental issue in South India, concerning biodiversity conservation and welfare of local communities.

In order to address these issues, this programme links up ecology and social sciences departments at IFP.

- Documentation of medicinal plants will be collected and organised in a database to understand their ecosystem, distribution and harvesting.
- Social sciences investigations will examine those environmentally related aspects as they pertain to the notion of space and to the local social and political dynamics.
- Spatial, social and political dynamics will be comprehended through the analysis of collection and marketing of medicinal plants, with a particular emphasis on the relationships between actors.
- This study on medicinal plants in South India is of interest for researchers and stakeholders to improve the conservation and forest management strategies.

MATERIALS AND METHODS

Surveys for building a regional database on medicinal plants, their uses and procurement will be conducted in three Southern Indian states (Karnataka, Kerala and Tamil Nadu). Data on the diveısity, abundance and distribution of medicinal plant species in various forest types will be gathered using the existing floristic and ecological database of FIP and additional field missions. Iconographic data on traits of species and parts used in different healing methods will be incorporated into the database.

In the initial phase, the analysis of medicinal plants' collection and marketing will be carried out in the landscape unit identified by FIP in. Data on spatial, social, economical, historical and political aspects of the medicinal plant procurement and marketing will be integrated to a Geographical Information System.

Medicinal plants, since times immemorial, have been used in virtually all cultures as a source of medicine. The widespread use of herbal remedies and healthcare preparations, as those described in ancient texts such as the Vedas and the Bible, and obtained from commonly used traditional herbs and medicinal plants, has been traced to the occurrence of natural products with medicinal properties.

The use of traditional medicine and medicinal plants in most developing countries, as a normative basis for the maintenance of good health, has been widely observed (UNESCO, 1996). Furthermore, an increasing reliance on the use of medicinal plants in the industrialised societies has been traced to the extraction and development of several drugs and chemotherapeutics from these plants as well as from traditionally used rural herbal remedies (UNESCO, 1998). Moreover, in these societies, herbal remedies have become more popular in the treatment of minor ailments, and also on account of the increasing costs of personal health maintenance. Indeed, the market and public demand has been so great that there is a great risk that many medicinal plants today, face either extinction or loss of genetic diversity.

BACKGROUND

Medicine, in several developing countries, using local traditions and beliefs, is still the mainstay of health care. As defined by WHO, health is a state of complete physical, mental, and social well being and not merely the absence of disease or infirmity. The practise of traditional medicine is widespread in China, India, Japan, Pakistan, Sri Lanka and Thailand. In China about 40% of the total medicinal consumption is attributed to traditional tribal medicines. In Thailand, herbal medicines make use of legumes encountered in the *Caesalpiniaceae*, the *Fabaceae*, and the *Mimosaceae*. In the mid-90s, it is estimated that receipts of more than US$2. 5 billion have resulted from the sales of herbal medicines. And, in Japan, herbal medicinal preparations are more in demand than mainstream pharmaceutical products.

Africa is a rich source of medicinal plants. Perhaps, the best known species is *Phytolacca dodecandra*. Extracts of the plant, commonly known as *endod*, are used as an effective molluscicide to control schistosomiasis (Lemma, 1991). Other notable examples are *Catharanthus roseus*, which yields anti-tumour agents such as vinblastine and vincristine; and *Ricinus communis*, which yields the laxative—castor oil. In Botswana, Lesotho, Namibia and South Africa, *Harpagophytum procumbens* is produced as a crude drug for export. Similarly, *Hibiscus subdariffa* is exported from Sudan and Egypt. Other exports are *Pausinystalia yohimbe* from Cameroon, Nigeria and Rwanda, which yields *yohimbine;* and *Rauwolfia vomitoria*, from Madagascar, Mozambique and Zaire, which is exploited to yield reserpine and ajmaline.

The use of medicinal plants like *Eupatorium perfoliatum* (bonest), *Podophyllum peltatum* (mayapple), and *Panax quinquefolium* (ginseng) in the USA has long been associated with the American Indians. These plants have also been appreciated and recognised for their aesthetic and ornamental value. In Central America medicinal plants have been widely used-by the *Maya* Indians in Mexico, the *Miskitos* and *Sumus* in Honduras and Nicaragua, the *Pech, Lencas,* and *Xicaques* in Honduras, the *Pipiles* in El Salvador, the *Talamancas* in Costa Rica, and the *Guaymis* and *Kunas* in Panama.

In Europe, some 1500 species of medicinal and aromatic plants are widely used in Albania, Bulgaria, Croatia, France, Germany, Hungary, Poland, Spain,

Turkey, and the United Kingdom. The Maltese islands constitute an apt example where medicinal plants are widely used in every day life as part of folk medicinal remedies (Lanfranco, 1992).

Issues

Traditional and folklore medicine bequeathed from generation to generation is rich in domestic recipes and communal practice. Encompassing concepts and methods for the protection and restoration of health, traditional medicine has served as a fount of alternative medicine, new pharmaceuticals, and healthcare products. The best known examples of traditional medicine, differing in concept and protocol, are well-developed systems such as acupuncture and ayurvedic medicine that have been widely used to conserve human health in China and India.

Developed countries, in recent times, are turning to the use of traditional medicinal systems that involve the use of herbal drugs and remedies. About 1400 herbal preparations are used widely, according to a recent survey in Member States of the European Union. Herbal preparations are popular and are of significance in primary healthcare in Belgium, France, Germany and the Netherlands. Such popularity of healthcare plant-derived products has been traced to their increasing acceptance and use in the cosmetic industry as well as to increasing public costs in the daily maintenance of personal health and well being. Examples of such beauty-oriented therapeuticals are skin tissue regenerators, anti-wrinkling agents and anti-age creams. Most dermaceuticals are derived from algal extracts that are rich in minerals and the vitamin B group. Skincare products such as skin creams, skin tonics, etc. derived from medicinal plants are grouped together as dermaceuticals. Also, amongst the poor, cures and drugs, derived from plants, constitute the main source of healthcare products.

Gorman (1992) drew attention to the power of Chinese folk medicinal potions in treating maladies from eczema and malaria to respiratory disorders. In the quest for new medicines to treat old and emergent diseases such as malaria and AIDS, attention is now being given to discovering the active ingredients encountered in the treasury of over 5, 000 Chinese herbs, plants and roots that have been used routinely and traditionally. *Quinghaosu* and *Chaihu* are two such examples. Whereas the former, called *artemisinin* and obtained from *Artemisia annua* is expected to yield, in the coming millennium, a potent new class of antimalarials, the latter, obtained from *Bupleurum chinense* and used as a popular remedy for hepatitis is the focus of intense research by the Japanese pharmaceutical industry. More recently, the biochemistry of *tianhuafen* or cucumber is being studied in the USA to decipher the identity of *compound Q*, an extract used in China and credited with remedial and relief properties in AIDS sufferers.

Medicinal plants are an integral component of ethnoveterinary medicine. Farmers and pastoralists in several countries use medicinal plants in the maintenance and conservation of the healthcare of livestock. Intestinal disorders in cows, in Mexico, are treated with herbal extracts of *Polakowskia tacacco*. Dietary supplements such as vitamin A in poultry feeds in Uganda are supplied through enrichments of amaranth (*Amaranthus sp.*). It is estimated that medicinal plants, for several centuries, have been widely used as a primary source of prevention and control of livestock diseases. In fact, interest of such use in the veterinary sector has resulted primarily from the increasing cost of livestock maintenance and the introduction of new technology in the production of veterinary medicines and vaccines.

McGee (1998), surveying the use of spice and their medicinal properties around the world, concluded that spices serve the adaptive purpose of reducing food-borne disease. In reviewing relevant texts ranging from the preservative properties of spices against food spoilage to the presence of antimicrobial substances that lay claim to the elimination of pathogenic organisms in food preparations, the case is made for a more objective analysis and study of the medicinal properties of spices *in victu* rather than *in victo*. A whole range of plant-derived dietary supplements, phytochemicals and pro-vitamins that assist in maintaining good health and combating disease are now being described as functional foods, nutriceuticals and nutraceuticals.

Despite the increasing use of medicinal plants, their future, seemingly, is being threatened by complacency concerning their conservation. Reserves of herbs and stocks of medicinal plants in developing countries are diminishing and in danger of extinction as a result of growing trade demands for cheaper healthcare products and new plant-based therapeutic markets in preference to more expensive target-specific drugs and biopharmaceuticals. Such concerns have stimulated positive legal and economic interest.

Issues concerning intellectual property rights, compensation for loss of finance-rich biodiversity resources, and the acquisition and safeguarding of traditional healthcare knowledge are no longer neglected. Bioprospecting of new drugs from medicinal plants and the exploitation of unprotected traditional knowledge in starting-up potentially new bioindustries are the focus of new monitoring measures. Such concerns that call for adherence to and observation of cultural and intellectual property rights have been addressed and enshrined in the *Chiang-Mai* and *Kari-Oca* Declarations. The first countries to seriously tackle these issues are China and India. Indeed, programmes dealing with medicinal plant conservation, cultivation, community involvement and sustainable development being initiated elsewhere, could benefit immensely from the Chinese and Indian experiences (World Bank, 1997).

Genetic biodiversity of traditional medicinal herbs and plants is continuously under the threat of extinction as a result of growth-exploitation, environment-unfriendly harvesting techniques, loss of growth habitats and unmonitored trade of medicinal plants.

Medicinal herbs, possessing penile potency properties and anti-cancer principles are the focus of smuggling to import markets in Germany, France, Switzerland, Japan, the U. K., and the U. S. A. The best known example, in recent times, is that of *tetu lakda* (*Nothadoytes foetida*). Commonly encountered in southern India and Sri Lanka, the herb is exploited as a source of anti-cancer drugs.

On the other hand, *Adonis vernalis*, extinct in Italy and the Netherlands, is an endangered species in Germany, Slovakia, Sweden and Switzerland. Fortunately, to safeguard against such practices and losses, guidelines and licensing concerning the use of such plants are provided for in the *Convention on International Trade Endangered Species of Wild Flora and Fauna* (CITES).

The industrial uses of medicinal plants are many. These range from traditional medicines, herbal teas, and health foods such as nutriceuticals to galenicals, phytopharmaceuticals and industrially produced pharmaceuticals. Furthermore, medicinal plants constitute a source of valuable foreign exchange for most developing countries, as they are a ready source of drugs such as quinine and reserpine; of galenicals like tinctures and of intermediates (e.g. diosgenin from *Discorea sp.)* in the production of semi-synthetic drugs. The world market for plant-derived chemicals – pharmaceuticals, fragrances, flavours, and colour ingredients, alone exceeds several billion dollars per year. Classic examples of phytochemicals in biology and medicine include taxol, vincristine, vinblastine, colchicine as well as the Chinese antimalarial-artemisinin, and the Indian ayurdevic drug-*forkolin*. Trade in medicinal plants is growing in volume and in exports. It is estimated that the global trade in medicinal plants is US$800 million per year.

The botanical market, inclusive of herbs and medicinal plants, in the USA, is estimated, at retail, at approximately US$1. 6 billion p. a. China with exports of over 120, 000 tonnes p. a., and India with some 32, 000 tonnes p. a. dominate the international markets. It is estimated that Europe, annually, imports about 400, 000 t of medicinal plants with an average market value of US$ 1 billion from Africa and Asia. A growing awareness of this new contributor to the foreign-exchange reserves of several national treasuries is beginning to emerge. To satisfy growing market demands, surveys are being conducted to unearth new plant sources of herbal remedies and medicines.

In several industrialised societies, plant-derived prescription drugs constitute an element in the maintenance of health. Medicinal plants are an integral component of research developments in the pharmaceutical industry. Such research focuses on the isolation and direct use of active medicinal constituents, or on the development of semi-synthetic drugs, or still again on the active screening of natural products to yield synthetic pharmacologically-active compounds. In Germany, for example, over 1500 plant species encountered in some 200 families and 800 genera have been processed into medicinal products. In South Africa, likewise, some 500 species are commercialised trade products. Today, Bulgaria, Germany and Poland are recognised as major exporters of plant-based medicinal products.

The development and commercialisation of medicinal plant-based bioindustries in the developing countries is dependent upon the availability of facilities and information concerning upstream and downstream bioprocessing, extraction, purification, and marketing of the industrial potential of medicinal plants. Absence of such infrastructure compounded by lack of governmental interest and financial support restricts the evolution of traditional herbal extracts into authenticated market products. Furthermore the absence of modernised socio-economic and public healthcare systems reinforces reliance of rural and lower-income urban populations on the use of traditional medicinal herbs and plants as complementary aids to routine pharmaceutical market products.

The prophylactic and therapeutic effects of plant foods and extracts in reducing cardiovascular disease has been reviewed (Walker, 1996). Non-nutrient phytochemicals are increasingly being recognised as potential health promoters in reducing the risks of cardiovascular disease and atherosclerosis. Prominent herbs identified were *Achillea millefolium* (yarrow), *Allium sativum* (garlic), *Convallaria majalis* (lily of the valley), *Crataegus laevigata* (hawthorn), *Cynara scolymus* (globe artichoke), *Gingko biloba* (gingko) and *Viburnum opulus* (cramp bark).

Saint-John's wort known as Johanniskrant in German for centuries has been used to treat people with mild and moderate depression without the side effects of Prozac. Widely sold in Germany and other European countries, and awaiting official approval by the US Food and Drug Administration, Saint-John's wort is being regarded as a serious rival to Prozac (Andrews, 1997).

Medicinal plants can make an important contribution to the WHO goal to ensure, by the year 2000, that all peoples, worldwide, will lead a sustainable socio-economic productive life. The Centre for Science and Technology of the Non-Aligned and other Developing Countries in India organised an international workshop on *Tissue Culture of Economic Plants* in April, 1994, as a means of using modern biotechnological techniques to nurture and conserve medicinal plants.

In late 1997, the World Bank, within the framework of the Global Environmental Facility, provided a US$ 4. 5 million grant for the *Sri Lanka Conservation of Medicinal Plants Project* which focuses on the conservation of medicinal plant populations, their habitats, and their sustainable use in Medicinal Plant Conservation Areas (MPCAs). Inventories with emphasis on the management, research and conservation of rare and endangered species of medicinal plants are the main programmes at MPCAs at Ritigala, Naula, Rajawaka, Kanneliya, and Bibile.

Aspects of policy and research concerning the cultivation of non-tropical and tropical medicinal plants and their genetic improvement; their conservation in botanical gardens; their storage in liquid nitrogen; their economic potential in international pharmaceutical trade; and their vulnerability to over-exploitation and extinction have been dealt with authoritatively. Moreover, such concerns and issues are addressed through a variety of programme activities and projects conducted, and promoted by several international, regional, and non-governmental organisations.

Concluding Remarks

Recent and renewed interest in medicinal plants coupled to developments in information technology has fuelled an explosion in the range and content of electronic information concerning medicinal plants as a re-emergent health aid. Bhat (1997) recently reviewed diverse sources of such information in traditional abstracting services as well as in a variety of online electronic databases. As a result of such developments, access to indigenous peoples and cultures concerning medicinal plants are greatly facilitated. Furthermore, the active participation of such natural custodians and practitioners of valuable knowledge is guaranteed in the generation of research focussing on screening programmes dealing with the isolation of bioactive principles and the development of new drugs.

IMPORTANCE OF MEDICINAL PLANTS

Important Medicinal Plants and their active constituents

Plant	Active principle activity	Pharmacological
1 *Rauvolfia serpentina*	Reserpine	Hypotensive
2 *Catharanthus roseus*	Ajmalicine	Vasodilator
	Vinblastine	Anticancer
	Vincristine	Anticancer

3 *Cassia angustifolia, Cassia acutifolia*	Sennosides	Laxative
4 *Plantago ovata*	Psyllium mucilage	laxative
5 *Glycyrrhiza glabra*	Glycyrrhizic acid	Antiinflammatory
6 *Berberis sp.*	Berberin	Antidiarrhoeal
7 *Digitalis lanata*	Digitoxin Lanatoside	Cardiotonic
8 *Taxus baccata*	Taxol	Anticancer
9 *Podophyllum emodi*	Podophyllotoxin	
Etoposide		
Tenoposide	Anticancer	
10 *Datura species, Hyocymus musticus, Duboisia myoporoides*	Hyoscine	
Syoscyamina		
Atropine	Parasympatholytic	
11 *Artemisai annua*	Artemisinin	Antimalarial
12 *Mappia foetida*	Camptothecine	Anticancer

Medicinal Plants used as Crude Extracts/Tinctures in Medicines

Botanical Name	**Common Name**
1 Belladonna	*Atropa belladonna*
2 Ipecac	*Cephaelis ipecacuanha*
3 Opium	*Papaver somniferum*
4 Henbane	*Hyoscyamus niger*
5 Stramonium	*Datura stramonium*
6 Liquorice	*Glycyrrhiza glabra*
7 Rhubarb	*Rheum officinale*
8 Podophyllum	*Podophyllium emodi*
9 Capscicum oleoresin	*Capsicum annum*
10 Digitalis	*Digitalis lanata, Digitalis purpurea*
11 Aloe	*Aloe vera*

Important Plant Products having great potential in Medicine

Plant Product	**Source**	**Pharmacological activity**
1 Valepotriates	*Valeriana wallichii*	Sedative, tranquilizer
2 Silymarin	*Silybum marianum*	Antihepatoxic
3 Podophyllotoxin (Etoposide/ tenoposide)	*Podophyllum emodi, P. pellatum*	Anticancer
4 Taxol	*Taxus baccata*	Anticancer
5 Guggul saponins	*Cormmiphora wiightii*	Hypolipidaemic
6 Artemisinin	*Artemisai annua*	Antimalarial

Some important medicinal plants suggested for cultivation :

Botanical name of the plant	Common
Aegle marmalos	Bilva (Hindi); Maredu (Telugu)
Glycyrrhiza glabra	Mulethi (Hindi); Athimadhuramu (Telugu)
Gmelina arborea	Gambhiri (Hindi); Gummadi (Telugu)
Mesua ferrea	Nagkesara (Hindi); Keearamu (Telugu)
Piper longum	Pipli (Hindi); Pippali (Telugu)
Picrorhiza kurroa	Kutki (Hindi); Katukarogani (Telugu)
Phyllanthus niruri	Jar-amla (Hindi); Nelausiri (Telugu)
Saraca indica	Ashoka (Hindi); Asokachettu (Telugu)
Swertia chirayata	Chirayata (Hindi); Nilavemyu (Telugu)
Andrographis paniculata	Kalmegha (Hindi); Nelavemu (Telugu)
Terminalia arjuna	Arjuna (Hindi); Tellamaddi (Telugu)
Valeriana wallichii	Tagar (Hindi)
Tinospora cordifolia	Gulancha (Hindi); Thippatheega (Telugu)
Asparagus racemosus	Shatavar (Hindi); Pillitheegalu (Telugu)
Plumbago zeylanica	Chita (Hindi); Chitramulamu (Telugu)
Conuniphora wightii	Guggul (Hindi, Telugu)
Boerhaavia diffusa	Punarnava, Sant (Hindi, Telugu)
Withania somnifera	Ashwagandha (Hindi, Telugu)
Bacopa monnieri	Brahmi (Hindi, Telugu)

Systems of Medicine

- There are mainly 3 systems of medicine practised in the world today. They are :

Modern System or Allopathy

- This system was developed in the Western countries. In this system drugs (tablets, capsules, injections, tonics etc.) are manufactured using synthetic chemicals and/or chemicals derived from natural products like plants, animals, minerals etc. This system also uses modern equipment for diagnosis, analysis, surgery etc.
- Medicines or drugs of this system is often criticised for its treatment of the symptoms rather than the cause of the disease, harmful side effects of certain drugs and for being out of reach of common/poor people due to the high cost of drugs and treatment.
- This system is used in all the countries of the world today.

Alternative Medicine or Traditional System

- Different countries of the world developed independently their own traditional systems of medicine using locally available materials like minerals and products of plants and animals.

- The World Health Organisation is giving considerable importance to these alternate medicine (as they act as alternative to allopathy) systems to provide Primary Health Care to millions of people in the developing countries.
- China developed the Chinese system of medicine, which is practised in China, Singapore, Taiwan, Japan and other countries.
- In Indonesia, Jamu and in South Africa, Zulu systems of herbal medicine are practised. The Unani or Tibb system was developed in the Middle Eastern Arab countries and is practised in India and in many countries.
- In India, Ayurveda (developed in North India), Siddha (developed in Tamil Nadu) and Nagarjuna (developed in Andhra Pradesh) systems of medicine were developed. Ayurveda is practised in Sri Lanka, Pakistan and Bangladesh also. Herbo-mineral is another traditional system used in India and other neighbouring countries.
- Drugs (balms, oils, pills, tonics, paste etc) are manufactured and marketed in these systems. The major advantage of these systems is that they are within the reach of the people, particularly rural poor.
- These systems are claimed to be pollution free, eco-freindly and have minimal or no harmful side effects. Ayurveda claims to cure the cause of the disease rather than the symptoms and is wholistic in its approach.
- In this system a disease is conceived as an imbalance in the systems of the body and the treatment aims at restoring the balance in the various systems of the body.

Folk Medicine

- The medicinal systems followed by various tribals/aborigins of different countries is popularly known as folk or tribal medicine.
- In the system, the "medicine man" or the "doctor" of the tribe who has the knowledge of treating diseases, keeps this knowledge as a closely guarded secret and passes it to the next generation by word of mouth.
- No written texts on these systems are available and different tribes follow different time tested methods. The treatment is often associated with lengthy and mystic rituals, in addition to prescription of drugs (decoctions, pastes, powders, oils, ashed materials etc.).
- Mostly locally available natural materials are used for the preparation of drugs, which are not commercially made and marketed. Generally speaking, folk medicine can also be regarded as a traditional system of medicine.
- The basic aim of all the above systems of medicine is to alleviate the sufferings of human beings and their domesticated animals.

- The knowledge of the traditional systems is undergoing close scientific scrutiny and is being increasingly incorporated into the modern system.

Other Systems

- Yoga, Acupressure, Acupuncture, Reiki, Magneto therepy, Pyramid therapy, Flower therapy, Homeopathy, Nature Cure or Naturopathy etc. are some of the other systems of medicine practised in different parts of the world today.

Utilization of Medicinal Plants

- The utility of medicinal plants has four major segments:
    - o Medicinal plants utilised in indigenous or traditional systems of medicines (ISM) -Ayurveda, Siddha, Unani and Homeopathy systems of medicines.
    - o OTC (over the country, non-prescription) items/products involving plant parts, extracts galenicals etc.
    - o Essential oils
    - o Phyto-pharmaceuticals or plants used in modern systems of medicine.

Medicinal plants used in Traditional Systems of Medicine

- Traditional medicine is widespread through the world and it comprises of those practices based on beliefs that were in existence, often for hundreds of years, before the development and spread of modern scientific medicines and which are still in use today.
- As its name implies, it is the part of tradition of each country which employs practices that have been handed down from generation to generation. Its acceptance by a population is largely conditioned by cultural factors and much of traditional medicine, therefore, may not be easily transferable from one culture to another.
- An important feature of traditional therapy is the preference of practitioner for compound prescriptions over single substance/drug as it is being held that some constituents are effective only in the presence of others.
- This renders assessment of efficacy and eventually identification of active principles as required in international standards much difficult than for simple preparation.
- In India, earlier the medicines used in indigenous systems of medicines were generally prepared by the practicing physicians by themselves, but now this practice has been largely replaced by the establishment of organised indigenous drug industries.

- It is estimated that at present there are more than 1, 00, 000 licensed registered practitioners of Ayurveda, Siddha, Unani medicine or Homeopathy.
- As far as the Ayurveda system of medicine is concerned, it does not rule out any substances being used as potential source of medicine.
- Presently about 1000 single drugs and 8000 compound drug formulations of recognised merit are in vogue.
- In fact reliable data on availability in different regions of country as well as supply and demand of medicinal plants used in production of indigenous medicines are not available.
- However, annual herbal drug market has been estimated around 2200 crores and is expected to reach up to 4000 crores by the year 2000.

Plants-parts, extracts and galenicals

- The direct utilisation of plant material is not only a feature of ISM in the developing world but also in developed countries like USA, UK, Germany etc., the various herbal formulations are sold on health food shops.
- Preparation of decoctions, tinctures, galenicals and total extracts of plants also form a part of many pharmacopoeias of the world.
- The current trend of medicinal plants based drug industry is to procedure standard extracts of plants as raw material.

Essential Oils from plants

- The essential oil industry was traditionally a cottage industry in India. Since 1947, a number of industrial companies have been established for large scale production of essential oils, oleoresins and perfumes.
- The essential oil from plants includes Ajowan oil, Eucalyptus oil, Geranium oil, Lavender oil, Palmarosa oil, Patchouli oil, Rose oil, Sandalwood oil, Turpentine oil and Vetiver oil.

Phyto-pharmaceuticals

- During the past decades, bulk production of plant based drugs has become an important segment of Indian pharmaceutical industry.
- Some of the phyto-pharmaceuticals which are produced in India at present include
  1. morphone,
  2. codeine,
  3. papaverine (*Papaver somniferum*),
  4. quinine,

5. quinidine,
6. cinchonine and cinchonidine (*Cinchona sp., C. calisaya, C. ledgeriana, C. officinais* and *C. succirubra*);
7. hyoscine,
8. hyoscyamine (*Hyocyamus niger* and *H. muticus*),
9. colchicine (*Gloriosa superbad, Colchicum luteum* and *Iphigenia stellata*),
10. cephaeline and emetin (*Cephalis ipacacuanha*),
11. sennosides A & B (*Cassia angustifolia* and *C. acutifolia*),
12. reserpine,
13. rescinnamine,
14. ajmalicine and ajmaline (*Rauvolfia serpentina*);
15. vinblastine and vincristine,
16. ajmalicine (raubacine) (*Catharanthus roseus*);
17. guggul lipid (*Commiphora wightii*);
18. taxol (*Taxus baccata*);
19. artemisinin (*Artemisai annua*) etc.

- For all these segments of drug, perfumery, flavouring and cosmetic industries, mostly the higher plants are one of the raw materials and comes from the natural resources i.e. forests through forest contractors employing local or tribal people or from the drug farms maintained by the growers of aromatic and medicinal plants.

2

Aromatic Plants

The aromatic plants possess odoriferous and volatile substances which occur as essential oils, gum exudate, balsam and oleoresin in one or more parts, viz. root, wood, bark, foliage, flower and fruit. The chemical nature of these aromatic substances may be due to a variety of complex the chemical compounds. Many of these aromatics are powerful germicides and have anti-bacterial properties, but the bulk of the produce finds use in perfumery and the food-flavouring industries. Amongst the two, the per-fumeru and allied industries consume much larger amounts of the natural fragrant material. According to the UN Word Statistics (1972), the annual world trade (excluding countries in eastern Europe) in essential oils and perfummery aromatics for 1969 was of the order of Rs 2250 million; also, a large quantity of the aromatic material of plant origin is utilized in cosmetics, toiletries and allied industries. Our current volume of foreign trade in the perfumery material, essential oils and aromatic compounds is around Rs 65 million and this amount accounts for 1. 6 per cent of the world trade. Some sixty-two types of essential oils come to the international market with a large and consistent demand. However, our treatment of the aromatic plants is confined to a few more important essential-oil crops grown in the country.

The methods employed to obtain aromatic substances from plants are classified into distillation, enfleurage, maceration, expression and solvent extraction. Expect in the case of flowers crops, such as jasmine and kewara in which the fragrant constituents are likely to be decomposed or destroyed, the essential oils are mostly obtained by distilling the produce; in fact, steam distillation is the oldest method of separation of essential oils. The perfumery material is filled in a large-galvanizediron still over a perforated netal grid. Water is filled in the still below the level of the grid so that it generates a low-pressure steam on heating to pass through the material. The water vapours carry with it the essential oil of the perfumery material. These vapours are passed through a condenser and collected in a vessel where the oil is ecanted with a separating-funnel.

A simple field distillation unit could be fabricated by a skilled blacksmith. For more efficient and quick distillation of the produce; " steam distillation" units are employed. These units are built on the same principle except that live steam at 40-100 1b pressure per inch is injected into the filling-still through perforated coils and the distillation is completed in a shorter period. It has the advantages of handling a larger quantity of the material, besides improving upon the recovery of the essential oil.

As stated earlier, the solvent-extraction method is employed for the extractors are of two types, viz. stationary and rotatory types, and low-bowling solvents, like petroleum either, alcohol or benzen, are used for extracting the odoriferous principles. The stationary type extractors consists of vertical cylinders provided with type extractors consists of vertical cylinders provided with perforated metal grids arranged horizontally around a central vertical shaft. The flower crop is charged over the grids which come into constant with the solvent periodically and the essential oil is removed in successive washings. The rotatory type consists of an iron drum which rotates on a horizontal axis. The interior of the drum is divided with a perforated metal partition of holding floers and the solvent is filled in the lower part of the extractor. While the drum moves, the solvent seeps through the perforations and drips back, so that the essential oil is washed out to the solvent. This extract is than distilled in a vacuum still at a low temperature to recover the disolvant. The floral concentrate, thus obtained, also contains some waxes and plant pigments which are removed by treating with warm alcohol. The filtered solution, so obtained, is either used as such, or is concentrated in vaccum into a viscous oil.

LEMON GRASS (Cymbopogon flexuosus Stapf.). It is a stemless perennial grass, found wild in the southern states of India. The leaves yield an aromatic oil, containing 75-85 per cent citral. The oil is used in soaps, cosmetics and disinfectants and is a raw material for manufacturing ions and vitamin A. The crop is grown on about 390, 000 ha in Kerals and about 90 per cent of the produce is exported, earning about Rs 10 million in foreign exchange annually.

The crop is grown mainly as a rain-fed crop on poor marginal lands. It is a hardy drought-resistant plant and is grown under a wided range of climatic conditions. Two types are recognized : (1) the red-stemmed grass is the true lemon-grass and a selection ' OD-19' made at the Lemon Grass Research Station, Oodakkali (Kerala) is recommended for high yield, (2) the white-stemmed (var. albscens) yields oil or low citral content. The crop is best propagated through seed raised in nurseries; 10kg of the seed produces enough seedlings for planting a hectare. About 2-month-old seedlings are planted in rows, 40 to 15x 10 cm apart, during rains and the first harvest is ready after 90 days. In Kerala, 3 harvests are obtained in the first year and 4 to 5 harvests during each of the 3 to 5 succeeding years; the crop is cut after every 60 to 65 days, except during the dry season. The fields are mannered liberally with ash and spent grass (obtained after the distillation of the oil); farmers seldom apply inorganic fertilizers. The herbage contains 0. 35% oil on fresh-weight basis. The grass yield ranges from 18 to 25 tonnes per hectare, giving 60-72 kg of oil.

CITRONELLA GRASS (Cymobopogon winteriaruns Jowitt). It is a stemless perennial grass. The oil is mainly used in soaps, Cosmetics, deodorants and mosquito-repellent creams. It is a recent introduction into India and its cultivation. mainly in the lower hills of Assam, in Karnataka and southern Gujrat, covers about 2, 000 hectares. A part of out requirement is still met by imports,

Java citronella is grown up to 1, 000 m above sea level on well-drained sandy-loanto clayey-loamy soils with pH varying from 5 to 7. 5 As a rainfed crop, it is propagated by using rooted slips, and is planted during the rainy season in rows, 60 to 45 cm x 45 to 30 cm apart, depending on the rate of growth and the soil fetility. Usually, the leafy portion is removed at planting during the monsoon season and the plants begin to tiller in 30 days after planting.

A healthy one-year-old clump yields 60 to 80 slips. The crop needs a large quantity of nitrogenous fertilizers, When grown on medium soils, it is given 60 kg of P, 40 kg of K and 20 kg of N per ha at planting, supplemented with 80 to 100 kg of N per hectare annually as top-dressing in 3 to 4 split doses. The crop is irrigated after every 10-15 days during the dry season and the first harvest is count 20 cm above the ground after 90 days of planting; usually 3 cuttings are obtained annually (4 under Assam conditions) for 3 to 5 year after planting.

CELERY (Apium graveolens Linn). Celery is a native of the Mediterranean region, introduced into India during late nineteenth century. India is now the principal grower (of the annual type) and exports large quantities of celery seeds (worth 17. 5 millions to the American and European markets. About 8000 ha is put under this crop, mainly in the Amritsar, Gurdaspur and Jallundhar districts of the Punjab State and to a smaller extent in the Saharanpur district of Uttar Pradesh. The clery seed is used in ground form as a dry seasoning powder and for the extraction of an oleoresin used to flavour a large variety of canned food products. The celery seed oil commands a larger market mainly in the confectionery industry. Whereas the bulk of celery seed is exported, a few local firms also produce its essential oil and olioresin on a small scale.

Celery is an erect, branchin herb, about 100 cm tall. it is a rabi crop which remains for 2 months in the nursery and for another 4 to 4 1/2 months in the field. Nursery is raised during early November. The seed-rate used is 2 kg. per hectare. The nursery-beds are kept moist and free from weeds through periodic irrigation followed by interculture. The seedlings grow up to 10 cm tall by the end of December and are ready for transplanting. The seedlings are usually planted 45 cm x 20 cm apart in early January in well-prepared fields, to which 30-50 tonnes of farmyard manure per ha is added during the preparatory tillage. On medium soils, about 80 Kg N, 40 Kg of P and 20 Kg of K per ha is applied to the crop; half of N along with the entire quantity of P and K is given to the rows at the time of planting and the remaining N is given as a top-dressing after one month. The crop requires 10-12 irrigations, each about 5 cm deep. Once established the crop requires 3 to 4 hoeings to keep down weeds. The plants bear flowers in umbels during early March and the fruits mature in late April. The Crop is harvested when about 80 per cent of the umbels begin to turn light brown. The harvested crop as stacked in the field for few days and is then threshed to obtain the seeds. The average grain yield ranges from 10 to 12 quintals per ha.

The celery (seed) on distillation yields to 2. 1 to 2. 3% of an essential oil containing selinene, d-limonene and sesquiterpenes. Oleoresin is prepared by using the method of the solvent extraction of the seeds. The seeds yields glycoside opiin. The crop remains remarkably free from pests and diseases.

Rose geranium (Pelargonium graveolens L'Herit) Pelargonium is a native of the hilly tracts of Cape Colony (South Africa). The highly aromatic 'Rose Geranium' is a hybrid (P. graveolens x P. radens), introduced by two Frenchmen-Earnest Sen and J. Priors in Yercaud in the Sheraroy Hills (Salem district) in Tamilnadu. It is now grown in a limited areas around Bangalore, Yercaud and in the Nilgiri Hills. The major world supplies of the oil come from Malagasy Republic. The oil of geranium has a refreshingly delicate rose-like aroma containing 66-78 per cent of alcohols calculated as geraniol. As such also, it itself is a perfume; it blends well with a wide range of floral and oriental perfumes. It is used for scenting oinments, pharmaceutical and tobacco products. It is suitable in a slightly alkaline medium and, therefore, it is widely used in the manufacture of high-grade soaps and cosmetic products. Our total annual production of the oil is around 12 tonnes and, therefore, a sizeable quantity of the oil is annually imported.

Two plant types of 'Rose Geranium' are recognized in India, Viz. the Algeriaan type from the slender plants, with dark pink flowers. It is less suitable for humid conditions; the other is Bourbin type which produces more leafy growth and bears light pink flowers. It is a perennial crop and about two to three harvests of leaves are taken annually in the second and third years. It can be grown as a catch crop in newly planted orchards.

'Rose Geranium' flourishes well in deep well-drained, preferably sandy loam to clayey-loam soils. It grows luxuriantly in a mild subtropical climate; locality receiving excessive heat in summer or very low temperatures in winter are unsuitable. The 'Rose Geranium' can withstand drought but its yield is reduced. It is raised in nursery during early spring from 8-15 cm long stem cutting each with 2 to 4 nodes. Sandy beds are preferred for the nursery to avoid excessive moisture which damages the young sprouts. Under a favourable day temperature of 10 to 15 degree Centigrade, about 80 per cent cuttings sproute in 3 weeks and are ready for field planting at 50 x 100 cm spacing with the onset of the monsoon rains in May-June. The field are brought to a fine tilth, are mixed with 45 tonnes of farmyard manure per hectare. In the Nilgiris the crop is given a basal application of a fertilizer mixture, containing 35, 45 and 17 kg of N, P and K per hectare; therefore, another 35 kg of N may be applied in two split applications annually. Initially, the crop is given 1 to 2 hoeings and weedings and the rows close up. The pruning of branches after the rains helps to induce bushy growth. The crop is irrigated at intervals of 10 to 15 days during summer depending upon the soils texture and the atmospheric humidity. Too moist or continued dry conditions lowers the crop yield. Generally, the first crop is obtained 6 to 8 months after planting and the average oil yields 8 kg; two or three crop are received in subsequent years, yielding 8 to 18 kg. of oil per hectare. In countries, e.g. Algeria and Malagasy Republic, the oil yields is reported to range from 30 to 35 kg. per hectare. The fresh leaves contain 0. 12 to 0. 2% (w/w) volatile oil and semi-dry or even dry leaves can be distilled. The oil improves in odour on ageing.

Fusarium sp. serious damages the geranium crop; the diseases is favoured by continued misty weather and excess soils moisture. The removal of diseased parts arrests the spread of the diseases and the spraying of the crop with 5% Bordeaux mixture periodically is recommended to control the diseases. However, when the roots are attacked, the plant dies and such infected plants should be pulled out along with the adhering soils and burnet.

PATCHOULI (Pogostemon cablin Benth) Patchouli is a native of humid Indo-Malayan tropics. The plant is small bushy herb which yields fragrant leaves containing a very sweet smelling oil. It is grown in small pockets mainly in Karnataka and Tamil Nadu. The oil of Patchouli is used to manufacture soap, cosmetics and incense and for imparting lasting oriental perfumery notes to many fancy products.

Two plants types of Patchouli are mainly recognized, viz. Jahore type which yields a poor leafy growth but produces a superior quality of oil; the other is Singapore type that gives more foliage and, therefore, more oil. It is a perennial crop, remaining in the field for about 3 years and gives 2 to 3 crops of leaves annually. It is a good catch crop for young orchards and can be raised as an intercrop in plantations where the over head shade is not heavy.

Patchouli requires deep, well-drained, fertile, slightly acidic soils, rich in humus; its growth is luxuriant in regions experiencing mild summer (24-280C), and a good rainfall ranging from 150 to 300 cm. Its sursery is raised in shade by planting 10-12 cm-long cuttings at 10 x 10 cm spacing during the rainy season and the beds are kept continuously moist. Under favourable conditions, about 85-90 per cent cutting per forth roots in a fortnight and they are ready for planting in the field in six to eight weeks at 90 x 90 cm spacing. The crop requires a liberal amount of organic matter and fertilizers; usually 10-12 tonnes of farmyard manure with 100 kg of P per ha is incorporated into the soil at the planting time, followed by 80 to 100 kg of N per hectare to the crop annually as top dressing in two split applications. The first crop is ready for harvesting in the next 4 to 6 months as indicated by the browning of the lower leaves, and the herbage is cut 10-25 cm below the apex in the morning hours. Usually, one or two growing branches are left unplucked to ensure a better growth of the succeeding harvest. The harvested leaves are dried in thin layers in sgade for 3-4 days and they develop their characteristic odour. Mature stalks are removed before distillation. Ageing improves the odour and the dry HA-77 leaves are therefore stored for a few months before distillation. A good crop stand yields about 2 tonnes of dry leaves (with 3 to 3. 5% oil) per annum, yielding about 50-60 kg of oil per hectare.

Golden nematode (Meloidogyne incognito) seriously damages this crop. No effective measure to control the nematode are known.

VETIVER OR KHUS (Vetiveria zizanioides (Linn Nash). Khus is a tall perennial grass found wild in the drier tracts of western India. Its spongy, much-branched fine root lets contain a fragrant oil, which is a perfume by itself. The dry aromatic roots are made into curtains, mats, fans, etc. to emit scented cool aroma when moistened. The oil is used as a valuable fixative for blending perfumes and socmetics. A large bulk of the oil is produced by distilling the wild-growing plants found in Bharatpur (Rajasthan), Musanagar, Biswan and Nawabganj etc. in western Uttar Pradesh. The cultivation of khus is scattered over small areas in the Trichur, Palghat, Kozikode, Wynad and Trivandrum district of Kerala, in the Tirunelvelly, Madhrai and Coimbatore districts of Tamil Nadu and in the kurnool and East Godavari districts of Andhra Pradesh.

In southern states, khus is grown as a rainfed crop in well-drained sandy-loam soils in moderately humid localities which received 100-200 cm of rainfall annually. However, a luxuriant growth of healthier roots is obtained from plants growing under warm and damp conditions on rich, partially inundated, masrshy land (Bharatpur). The field are laid out into beds of convenient size and 15-20 cm-long rooted slips are planted. With the onset of the monsoon rains on both the sides of the ridges, made 45 cm apart. The planting of 2 to 3 slips is done in spring in pits when the crop is raised under irrigation. The crop is given 10-12 tonnes of farmyard manure or compost at planting, supplemented with ash and groundnutcake or ammonium sulphate, one month after planting to stimulate growth.

Khus is a 12 to 18 month crop and the roots are dug out during dry months before autumn. The aerial parts are first cut at a height of 15 to 20 cm and are removed, the clumps are then dug out and beaten. The soil is further dug out up to a depth of one metre to remove the remaining rootlets. The roots are light to yellowish brown containing usually 0. 6 to 0. 8 per cent of dark brown viscous, persistently fragrant oil. The yield is 3 to 5 tonnes of fresh root, yielding about 20 kg of oil per hectare.

JASMINE. Among the perfume yielding jasmines, juhi (Jasminum curiculatum Vahl) and chameli (J officinale Linn) are commonly used for producing attars which sell at fancy prices. Jasmine ' concrete' and absolutes' are used to impart a gentle pleasing aroma to innumerable high-grade preparations. In the Western countries, Spanish (alsocalled French) jasmine (J. officinale Linn var grandiflorum Bailey) is largely cultivated; it has 7 to 11 leaflets and the flower bud has a dull creamy to punish spot on the posterior most petal. A high yelding clone of the Spanish jasmine has been recently developed at the Tamil Nadu Agricultural University, Coimbatore. It blooms from March to December and is reported to yield about 12 tonnes of fresh flowers per hectare annually against 1. 6 to 3 tonnes of flowers obtained from the Spanish jasmine in India. The crop remains in the field for 10 to 15 years.

The jasmines prefer well drained, rich sandy-loam to clayey-loam soils and remain in loom longer in a mild climate; the var. grandiflorum is more sensitive to fros. It is raised from 20 cm long stem cutting prepared from near mature wood and planted in deep pits at 1. 5 x 1 m spacing during the rainy season. The growing plants are pruned during January February and July to induce lateral branching and flowering, and are given farmyard manure liberally. The plantation needs fortnightly irrigation during dry months. Picking is done during the early morning hours and the percentage recovery of the concrete ranges from 0. 24 to 0. 38 by using the solvent extraction method. Fresh flowers lose their fragrance soon, and it is essential that the solvent extraction apparatus as available at the site where the jasmine plantation is raised for perfumery aromatics.

KEWARA (Pandanus odoratissimus Linn) Kewara is a large indigenous shrub, 3 to 6 m tall, bearing white or creamy dioecious flowers including its enclosing spathe contains a fragrant oil. The kewara attar and kewara water are commonly used at ceremonial functions in perfuming aerated waters, other drinks and confectionery products. Most of the cultivation is confined to the Ganjam district (400 ha) in Orissa where it is drains and ponds. The plant thrives in clayey loam soil in the tropical climate, usually receiving heavy rainfall.

Kewara is propagated from shoots, branches and leaves which readily from roots during the rainy season. It bears flowers in the fourth or fifth year and has an economic life of 20 years. The crops needs no special care, except periodic pruning. The flowers are borne from June to September. A plant may produce 15 to 40 flowers in a season. A flower takes 15 days to mature and grows grammes. The blossom contains 0. 1 to 0. 3 per cent oil. The attar is mosly produced over sandalwood oil or paraffin base.

MODERN EVIDENCE FOR THE ANTISEPTIC POWERS OF ESSENTIAL OILS

Towards the end of the 19th century, the first acknowledged research to prove the antiseptic properties of essential oils was that undertaken by Chamberland. This was followed early in the 20th century by Cavel's research into the individual effects of 35 essential oils on microbial cultures in sewage. The most effective oil in terms of the quantity required to render inactive 1000 ml of culture was found to be thyme (0.7 ml). Two other well-known oils showing high efficacy were sweet orange (1.2 ml, 3rd) and peppermint (2.5 ml, 9th). The antiseptic power of several oils has now been proved to be many times greater than that of phenol. Certain essential oils have also been shown to be effective against different bacteria, e.g lemon, which is one of the best in its antiseptic and bactericidal properties, neutralizing both the typhus bacillus and Staphylococcus aureus in a matter of minutes. Cinnamon kills the typhus bacillus even when diluted to 1 part in 300.

Professor Griffon, a member of the French Academy of Pharmacy, made up a blend of seven essential oils (cinnamon, clove, lavender, peppermint, pine, rosemary and thyme) to study their antiseptic effect on the surrounding air when sprayed from an aerosol; all the staphylococci and moulds present were destroyed after 30 minutes.

The bacteriological approach of aromatherapy is an extremely complex field of the utmost interest, opening the way to the ecological understanding and management of the different colonies and flora that live in cohabitation—or at war—within us. Allopathic medicine has begun to realise that the misuse of antibiotics leads to numerous side-effects and sometimes results in chronic disastrous conditions (i.e. systemic candidosis) that could have been avoided if medical aromatherapy had been implemented in due time.

Today, the properties of herb volatile oils are researched in many centres throughout the world.

WIDE-RANGING APPLICATION

Essential oils can be put to a multitude of uses both in general practice and in hospitals, as this quote from Dr. J. Valnet illustrates: The doctor who is familiar with essential oils can use them to treat a whole range of infections—pulmonary, hepatic, intestinal, urinary, uterine, rhinopharyngeal and cutaneous (infected wounds and suppurating dermatoses). The use of these oils usually produces satisfactory results, provided they have been prescribed wisely and that, in the case of certain long-standing complaints, the treatment is followed for a long enough period. Aromatic therapy can neutralise enteritis, colitis and putrid fermentations, and can relieve chronic bronchitis and pulmonary tuberculosis. The colon bacillus cannot resist essential oils.

Orthodox medicine currently uses plant material to help cure diseases which previously had a high death rate. Twenty years ago, four out of every five children with leukaemia lost their lives; nowadays four out of five are returned to health with the aid of vincristine and vinblastine, derivatives of the rosy periwinkle—a plant used for hundreds of years by tribal healers as a medicine. The snakeroot plant from India is now used in the Western world to treat hypertension; digitalis, for heart conditions, is produced from the humble foxglove and the well-known rhododendron is used in the treatment of fatigue. 'Plants are an intrinsic part of natural medicine, and not even the most orthodox doctor can get by without them; indeed they represent the link between the natural and the orthodox, the traditional and the ultra-new'.

Phytotherapy is the name increasingly given to the use of the whole, or part, of the plant for medicinal purposes. Aromatherapy and aromatology (similar to aromatherapy but including intensive and internal uses) are branches of this, utilizing only the essential oils produced by distillation and citrus oils produced by expression. These are simple to use and administer, yet can compete with the steroids and antibiotics used in allopathic medicine today without the body's defence mechanism becoming exhausted or tolerance developing to them.

The basic reason which accounts for the diversity of conception and application of aromatherapy lies in the very nature of the aromatic substance. Lending itself to easy cutaneous penetration, being endowed with the capacity to influence the mind through its powerful impact upon the olfactive sense, and owing multiple and strong pharmacological properties to its highly active molecular components, it was natural for the aromatic substance to find developments in so many areas.

POWERFUL HEALING AGENTS

Many plant extracts used in the production of conventional medicines are, like the foxglove, poisonous and therefore exceptionally low doses are employed. Some essential oils are also toxic when used incorrectly and the most powerful of these are not normally available to aroma therapists. Essential oils are concentrated and intensely energetic in their effects, so very little is needed (even of those in general use) for successful treatment—dilutions generally being in the range 0.05-3 percent, depending on the oil used. Apart from the difference in the intensity of the aroma, no apparent benefit is gained from higher concentrations, particularly where the problem is an emotional one, although neat oils are used in certain medical conditions and aromatology.

THEIR MODE OF ACTION

It cannot yet be proved exactly how they work, but research and extensive anecdotal evidence exists to prove that they do work. In the distant past, essences have been used to heal wounds, inhibit the decay of flesh (as in mummification) and reduce the spread of infection (as in the time of the Black Death)—all without anyone knowing how they worked, just as the humble aspirin was in use for many years before anyone knew its mode of action.

Bios is the Greek word for life and essential oils may be classed as probiotic (for life), as opposed to antibiotic (against life). To illustrate this point, antibiotics kill not only harmful bacteria, but also the beneficial flora that we need to keep us healthy, leaving the body in a weakened state. Carefully selected essential oils kill only the bacteria inimical to the successful functioning of the body. Some essential oils also possess antiviral and fungicidal qualities. 'A serious condition obviously authorises the use of antibiotics, and in high doses; but one should be aware that the price of a cure may be a permanent disability'.

USER-FRIENDLY

Natural, whole essential oils can be used on living tissue with minimal unwanted effects (unlike some synthetic drugs, however successful these may be against their intended targets). Also, the human body accustoms itself to the effects of chemical synthetics, leading to escalating doses. This has not been found to be the case with essential oils, which retain their effectiveness in repeated applications and can in fact strengthen the living tissue while killing off the unwanted bacteria.

QUANTITIES OF ESSENTIAL OILS USED

Tens of thousands of tonnes of essential oils are used by the food and perfume industries with the food industry being the largest user. It is important to realise that the total amount of essential oil used by the aromatherapy profession is extremely small compared with these industries, and this contributes to the difficulties of obtaining high quality, pure, natural oils Some oils which could be beneficial when used in aromatherapy are not generally supplied by distillers because they are not required by the giant users. Fortunately, however, a small number of independent distillers produce essential oils solely for aromatherapy use, although such products tend to be more expensive.

ECONOMY OF USE

Compared with the very high price of drugs (perhaps due to the tremendous research and development costs) essential oils are extremely inexpensive—a factor which should interest those in charge of public health funds. Not only that, they are pleasant to use for both patient and career. In many hospitals and hospices they are used not only to improve the quality of a patient's life but in waiting rooms to relieve the anxiety of relatives and friends. More specifically, they can be used in place of secondary drugs, which might be prescribed to counteract iatrogenic effects of the primary drugs being taken. They have been found to aid relaxation effectively, both pre- and post-operatively, to regenerate tissue in cases of severe burns and inflammation, and to relieve pain in cases of rheumatoid arthritis. They have helped to improve the quality of life for the terminally ill, and they have also found important uses in maternity care.

AREAS OF USE

Essential oils are used extensively by aroma therapists and aromatologists to improve or uplift a patient's state of mind. The effect of the attitude of mind on a person's health is being recognized more and more and essential oils can play an important part here. Florence Nightingale said 'what nursing has to do... is to put the patient in the best condition for nature to act upon him', reinforcing the ancient tag medicus cura, natura sanat—the doctor treats, nature cures.

By far the majority of essential oil users are outside the medical profession, some people using them merely on instruction from one of the many books written for the general public on the subject. They are simple to use and it should come as a relief to GPs that minor everyday ailments such as a sore throat or a winter cold, and even some more serious problems like bronchitis, sinusitis and rheumatism, can be treated in the home easily and successfully, leaving the doctor's time free for the cases requiring expert knowledge.

All this is achievable by anyone, without professional medical skills. However, in France (from where aromatherapy was introduced to the UK) doctors prescribe essential oils for internal use in capsules or in drops diluted in alcohol, or in suppositories and pessaries. They are used externally in dressings, fumigations, inhalations, ointments and in foot, hand or complete baths. The original concept of aromatherapy in England, as introduced by Mme Maury, was to use the essential oils in massage only— suitably diluted in a fixed vegetable oil. This unfortunately led to the belief that this is all there is to aromatherapy, and the authors are actively trying to correct this image. It needs the medical profession not only to take an interest but also to use its professional skills to utilize these precious commodities to their fullest capabilities in order to bring the benefits of this aromatic therapy to the hospitals of the world in the 21st century.

The subject of aromatherapy involves pharmacy and farming, botany and bodies, medicine and chemistry, toxicity and safety—all so intertwined and interconnected that it is scarcely possible to disentangle the ramifications for the purpose of setting them down without some repetition and much cross-referral.

SOME IMPORTANT GRASS AS AROMATIC PLANT

Lemon Grass (Cymbopogon Flexuosus Stapf.)

It is a stemless perennial grass, found wild in the southern states of India. The leaves yield an aromatic oil, containing 75-85 per cent citral. The oil is used in soaps, cosmetics and disinfectants and is a raw material for manufacturing ions and vitamin A. The crop is grown on about 390,000 ha in Kerals and about 90 per cent of the produce is exported, earning about Rs 10 million in foreign exchange annually.

The crop is grown mainly as a rain-fed crop on poor marginal lands. It is a hardy drought-resistant plant and is grown under a wided range of climatic conditions. Two types are recognized:

1. The red-stemmed grass is the true lemon-grass and a selection 'OD-19' made at the Lemon Grass Research Station, Oodakkali (Kerala) is recommended for high yield,
2. The white-stemmed (var.albscens) yields oil or low citral content. The crop is best propagated through seed raised in nurseries; 10kg of the

seed produces enough seedlings for planting a hectare. About 2-month-old seedlings are planted in rows, 40 to 15x 10 cm apart, during rains and the first harvest is ready after 90 days. In Kerala, 3 harvests are obtained in the first year and 4 to 5 harvests during each of the 3 to 5 succeeding years; the crop is cut after every 60 to 65 days, except during the dry season. The fields are manured librally with ash and spent grass (obtained after the distillation of the oil); farmers seldom apply inorganic fertilizers. The herbage contains 0.35 percent oil on fresh-weight basis. The grass yield ranges from 18 to 25 tonnes per hectare, giving 60 - 72 kg of oil.

Citronella Grass (Cymobopogon Winteriaruns Jowitt)

It is a stemless perennial grass. The oil is mainly used in soaps, Cosmetics, deodorants and mosquito-repellent creams. It is a recent introduction into India and its cultivation. mainly in the lower hills of Assam, in Karnataka and southern Gujrat, covers about 2,000 hectares. A part of out requirement is still met by imports

Java citronella is grown up to 1,000 m above sea level on well-drained sandy-loanto clayey-loamy soils with pH varying from 5 to 7.5 As a rainfed crop, it is propagated by using rooted slips, and is planted during the rainy season in rows, 60 to 45 cm x 45 to 30 cm apart, depending on the rate of growth and the soil fetility. Usually, the leafy portion is removed at planting during the monsoon season and the plants begin to tiller in 30 days after planting. A healthy one-year -old clump yields 60 to 80 slips. The crop needs a large quantity of nitrogenous fertilizers, When grown on medium soils, it is given 60 kg of P, 40 kg of K and 20 kg of N per ha at planting, supplemented with 80 to 100 kg of N per hectare annually as top-dressing in 3 to 4 split doses. The crop is irrigated after every 10-15 days during the dry season and the first harvest is count 20 cm above the ground after 90 days of planting; usually 3 cuttings are obtained annually (4 under Assam conditions) for 3 to 5 year after planting.

Celery (Apium Graveolens Linn)

Celery is a native of the Mediterranean region, introduced into India during late ninteenth century. India is now the principal grower (of the annual type) and exports large quantities of celery seeds (worth 17.5 millions to the American and European markets. About 8000 ha is put under this crop, mainly in the Amritsar, Gurdaspur and Jallundhar districts of the Punjab State and to a smaller extent in the Saharanpur district of Uttar Pradesh. The clery seed is used in ground form as a dry seasoning powder and for the extraction of an oleoresin used to flavour a large variety of canned food products. The celery seed oil commands a larger market mainly in the confectionery industry. Whereas the bulk of celery seed is exported, a few local firms also produce its essential oil and olioresin on a small scale.

Celery is an erect, branchin herb, about 100 cm tall. it is a rabi crop which remains for 2 months in the nursery and for another 4 to 4 1/2 months in the field. Nursery is raised during early November. The seed - rate used is 2 kg. per hectare. The nursery - beds are kept moist and free from weeds through periodic irrigation followed by interculture. The seedlings grow up to 10 cm tall by the end of December and are ready for transplanting. The seedlings are usually planted 45 cm x 20 cm apart in early January in well - prepared fields, to which 30-50 tonnes of farmyard manure per ha is added during the preperatory tillage. On medium soils, about 80 Kg N, 40 Kg of P and 20 Kg of K per ha is applied to the crop; half of N along with the entire quantity of P and K is given to the rows at the time of planting and the remaining N is given as a top - dressing after one month. The crop requires 10-12 irrigations, each about 5 cm deep. Once estalished the crop requires 3 to 4 hoeings to keep down weeds. The plants bear flowers in umbels during early March and the fruits mature in late April. The Crop is harvested when about 80 per cent of the umbels begin to turn light brown. The harvested crop as stacked in the field for few days and is then threshed to obtain the seeds. The average grain yield ranges from 10 to 12 quintals per ha.

The celery (seed) on distillation yields to 2.1 to 2.3 percent of an essential oil containing selinene,d-limonene and sesquiterpenes. Oleoresin is prepared by using the method of the solvent extraction of the seeds. The seeds yields glycoside opiin. The crop remains remarkably free from pests and diseases.

Patchouli (Pogostemon Cablin Benth)

Patchouli is a native of humid Indo-Malayan tropics. The plant is small bushy herb which yields fragrant leaves containing a very sweet smelling oil. It is grown in small pockets mainly in Karnataka and Tamil Nadu. The oil of Patchouli is used to manufacture soap, cosmetics and incense and for imparting lasting oriental perfumery notes to many fancy products.

Two plants types of Patchouli are mainly recognized, viz. Jahore type which yields a poor leafy growth but produces a superior quality of oil; the other is Singapore type that gives more foliage and, therefore, more oil. It is a perennial crop, remaining in the field for about 3 years and gives 2 to 3 crops of leaves annually. It is a good catch crop for young orchards and can be raised as an intercrop in plantations where the over head shade is not heavy.

Patchouli requires deep, well-drained, fertile, slightly acidic soils, rich in humus; its growth is luxuriant in regions experiencing mild summer (24-280C), and a good rainfall ranging from 150 to 300 cm. Its sursery is raised in shade by planting 10-12 cm-long cuttings at 10 x 10 cm spacing during the rainy season and the beds are kept continuously moist. Under favourable conditions, about 85-90 per cent cutting per forth roots in a fortnight and they are ready for planting in the field in six to eight weeks at 90 x 90 cm spacing. The crop requires a liberal amount of organic matter and fertilizers; usually 10-12 tonnes of farmyard manure with 100 kg of P per ha is incorporated into the soil at the planting time, followed by 80 to 100 kg of N per hectare to the crop annually as top dressing in two split appications. The first crop is ready for harvesting in the next 4 to 6 months as indicated by the browning of the lower leaves, and the herbage is cut 10-25 cm below the apex in the morning hours. Usually, one or two growing branches are left unplucked to ensure a better growth of the succeeding harvest. The harvested leaves are dried in thin layers in sgade for 3-4 days and they develip their characteristic odour. MAture stalks are removed before distillation. Ageing improves the odour and the dry HA-77 leaves are therefore stored for a few months before distillation. A good crop stand yields about 2 tonnes of dry leaves (with 3 to 3.5 percent oil) per annum, yielding about 50-60 kg of oil per hectare.

Golden nematode (Meloidogyne incognito) seriously damages this crop. No effective meaasure to control the nematode are known.

Vetiver or Khus (Vetiveria Zizanioides (Linn Nash)

Khus is a tall perennial grass found wild in the drier tracts of western India. Its spongy, much-branched fine root lets contain a fragrant oil, whcih is a perfume by itself. The dry aromatic roots are made into curtains, mats, fans, etc. to emit scented cool aroma when moistened. The oil is used as a vlauable fixative for blending perfumes and socmetics. A large bulk of the oil is produced by distilling the wild-growing plants found in Bharatpur (Rajasthan), Musanagar, Biswan and Nawabganj etc. in western Uttar Pradesh. The cultivation of khus is scattered over small areas in the Trichur, Palghat, Kozikode, Wynad and Trivandrum district of Kerala, in the Tirunelvelly, Madhrai and Coimbatore districts of Tamil Nadu and in the kurnool and East Godavari districts of Andhara Pradesh

In southern states, khus is grown as a rainfed crop in well-drained sandy-loam soils in moderately humid localities which received 100-200 cm of rainfall annually. However, a luxuriant growth of healthier roots is obtained from plants growing under warm and damp conditions on rich, partially inundated, masrshy land (Bharatpur). The field are laid out into beds of convenient size and 15-20 cm-long rooted slips are planted. With the onset of the monsoon rains on both the sides of the ridges, made 45 cm apart. The planting of 2 to 3 slips is done in spring in pits when the crop is raised under irrigation. The crop is given 10-12 tonnes of farmyard manure or compost at planting, supplemented with ash and groundnutcake or ammonium sulphate, one month after planting to stimulate growth.

Khus is a 12 to 18 month crop and the roots are dug out during dry months before autumn. The aerial parts are first cut at a height of 15 to 20 cm and are removed, the clumps are then dug out and beaten. The soil is further dug out up to a depth of one metre to remove the remaining rootlets. The roots are light to yellowish brown containing usually 0.6 to 0.8 per cent of dark brown viscous, persistently fragrant oil. The yield is 3 to 5 tonnes of fresh root, yielding about 20 kg of oil per hectare.

Jasmine

Among the perfume yielding jasmines, juhi (Jasminum curiculatum Vahl) and chameli (J officinale Linn) are commonly used for producing attars which sell at fancy prices. Jasmine ' concrete' and absolutes' are used to impart a gentle pleasing aroma to innumerable high-grade perparations. In the Western countries, Spanish (alsocalled French) jasmine (J. officinale Linn var grandiflorum Bailey) is largely cultivated; it has 7 to 11 leaflets and the flower bud has a dull creamy to punish spot on the posterior most petal. A high yelding clone of the Spanish jasmine has been recently developed at the Tamil Nadu Agricultural University, Coimbatore. It blooms from March to December and is reported to yield about 12 tonnes of fresh flowers per hectare annually against 1.6 to 3 tonnes of flowers obtained from the Spanish jasmine in India. The crop remains in the field for 10 to 15 years.

The jasmines prefer well drained, rich sandy-loam to clayey-loam soils and remain in loom longer in a mild climate; the var. grandiflorum is more sensitive to fros. It is raised from 20 cm long stem cutting prepared from near mature wood and planted in deep pits at 1.5 x 1 m spacing during the rainy season. The growing plants are pruned during January February and July to induce lateral branching and flowering, and are given farmyard manure liberally. The plantation needs fortnightly irrigation during dry months. Picking is done during the early morning hours and the precentage recovery of the concrete ranges from 0.24 to 0.38 by using the solvent extraction method. Fresh flowers lose their fragrance soon, and it is essential that the solvent extraction apparatus as available at the site where the jasmine plantation is raised for perfumery aromatics.

Kewara (Pandanus Odoratissimus Linn)

Kewara is a large indigenous shrub, 3 to 6 m tall, bearing white or creemy dioecious flowers including its enclosing spathe contains a fragrant oil. The kewara attar and kewara water are commonly used at ceremonial functions in perfuming aerated waters, other drinks and confectionery products. Most of the cultivation is confined to the Ganjam district (400 ha) in Orissa where it is drains and ponds. The plant thrives in clayey loam soil in the tropical climate, usually receiving heavy rainfall.

Kewara is propagated from shoots, branches and leaves which readily from roots during the rainy season. It bears flowers in the fourth or fifth year and has an economic life of 20 years. The crops needs no special care, except periodic pruning. The flowers are borne from June to September. A plant may produce 15 to 40 flowers in a season. A flower takes 15 days to mature and grows grammes. The blossom contains 0.1 to 0.3 per cent oil. The attar is mosly produced over sandalwood oil or paraffin base.

Davana (Artemisia Pallens Wall)

It is a small (50 cm tall) annual indigenous herb with divided pluish green fragrant leaves. The oil of the herb is prized in perfumery for its sweet, persistent fruity fragrance. It is cultivated on a limited scale in karnataka for making bouquets and producing oil. It is a 4 month rabi crop raised in fertile well drained red loamy soils under equable climate receiving mild winter rains and with clear sunny weather ar maturity. Seeds are small (about 6000 g) and are kept in a moist piece of cloth for 1-2 lays for germination. The sprouted seed are thinly broadcast in the nursery in early November abd the seedlings establish themselves in 7-10 days. Five week old seedlings are planted in the field. The crop is given mainly their usual height in 10 weeeks afterplanting. The crop is harvested on bright sunny days and the harvested herb is air dried. The air dried herb is chopped into 3 to 4 pieces and distilled at prssure of 2 kg per sq. cm for 8 to 12 hours. The yield of fresh herbage is about 30 tonnes per ha. The harbage loses about four fifths of its moisture on drying; the averageoil content of the dry herb is 0.2 per cent. Thus 10 to 12 kg of brownish viscous oil is attained from one hectare. Its quantity improves with age.

Henna or Mehandi (Lawsonia Inermis Linn)

It is a persnnial hedge plant, native to North Africa. It is cultivated in the Pali, Sojat abd Nagor districts of Rajasthan and the adjoining districts of Gurgaon and Faridabad in Haryana. The crop is grown in sandy loam to loamy soils in the hot and dry climate on marginal land. Two varities are known, viz. Hinna (odorous) and Rajni (more colouring). A part of the produce is exported.

Mehndi is raised through seeds as well as through cuttings; the former method is preferred. The seeds have a hard coat and are kept under a moist piece of cloth for 8-15 days till they sprout (the average germination being 20 per cent). The sprouted seeds are mixed with fine sand and sown broadcast in a well prepared nursery during March. The seedbeds are kept moist and free from weeeds. The seedlings grow 20-30 cm tall in the next 3 months and are transplanted in wet field during the monsoon season at 15 x 30 cm or 30 x 30 cm spacing. The land is given 40 tonnes of farmyard manure and 40 kg of N per ha at planting and a similar quantity thereafter in 2 split doses annually to boost vegetative growth.

The field are bunded during the rainy season to conserve moisture. Usually the plants in third year begin to yield the leaf crop which continues to start economic yields for the nest 25 years or so. Normally, 2 harvests are taken branches are cut near the ground level and dried, preferable in shade. The dry branches are beaten on yield under rain fed conditions is 1 tonne per ha; higher yields up t 2.5 tonnes per ha are obtained when raised as an irrigated crop. Termites, ants and mites damage the crop; the dusting of the crop with BHC (10 percent) is recommended as a preventive measure.

Sweet Flag or Bach (Acorus Calamus L)

It is a perennial indigenous undershrub which inhabits stagnant pools and shallow creaks all over the country. Its long aromatic rhizomes contain an aromatic oil (Ascerone 82 percent) used for lending oriental notes in perfumery; the oil has germicidal properties and is used in insecticidal formulations. It is a 10 month crop cultivated in clayey to clayey loam soils on about 500 ha confined to the koratgere Taluk of the Tumkar district in Karnataka. Field are puddled with 40 tonnes if farmyard manure or with sullage and bunded like rice field for impounding water. The growing tops of the plants obtained from the previous crop are usually planted in March - April in soft mud at 30 x 30 cm spacing and the field are flooded with 5 cm deep water. As the crop grows, the depth of water in the field is raised to 10 cm till about a month before harvest. The crop is given weeding almost every month for the first 4 to 5 months when the plants close the rows and produce a thick cover. Fertilizers are seldomused; some farmers apply 40 kg of N in 2 splits 30 and 60 days after planting. The leaf tips begin to turn yellow as the crop matures. The rhizomes are then dug out. The rhizomes lie mostly near the surface and grow 30 to 50 cm long. They are washed, cut into 6 to 10 cm long pieces and rubbed with hessain to remove the leafy scales and fibrous roots before drying them in the sun. The crop yield ranges from 2.5 to 4 tonnes of dry rhizomes per ha. The produce can be stored for a long period.

Linaloe (Bursera Delpechianum Boiss Ex. Engl)

It is a small Mexican tree whose wood (7-9 percent) and berries (3 percent) yield a sweet smelling essential oil on steam distillation. The characteristic odour of the oil due to the presence of 35-44 percent of easter (linalyll acetate) and 32-48 per cent of free alcohols (linalool) resembling the odour of lavender. The oil is used in the manufacture of high quality soaps and cosmetic products.

Linaloe is a dioecious plant which grows about 6 meters tall abd 1 meter in girth at 20 years of age. It sheds its leaves at the commencement of winter and gives out new leaves and flowers in April. The berries ripen in Aughst September and are collected before dehiscence. In its natural habitat, the plant grows in tropical serub forests on dry eroded land and is sensitive to frost and water logging. Its growth is better on fertile forest land. Spring rains benefit the crop. Cutting, about 0.5 m in length and 1 cm in diameter, are made from the female mother plants during February March and planted in pots, baskets or polythene bags in a nursery in shade. It sprouts in 3-4 weeks and, as such, is planted in pits during the rainy season.

About 300 plants are planted per ha. and they need irrigation in the succeeding summer season. The plants bear flowering twigs at 3 or 4 years of age. The flowering twigs are clipped. In the sixth year, the plants develops a crown spread of about 2m and commences giving the commercial crop. ipe beries are collected during automn and dried in shade. The dry fruits split in two, exposing the kernels. The essential oil is confined to the husk of the fruit. The dry berries can be stored for long and distilled at convenience. They yield 2.5 to 3 per cent oil on fresh weight basis. The yield of oil is around 20 kg/ha from the sixth year onards for a growing life span of about 50 years

Lemon Gum (Eucalyptus Citriodora Hook)

It is an Australian tree, about 25 m tall, with a clean silvery green trunk and strongly-scented narrow leaves. The plant is coppiced at a height of 90 cm to get a larger yield of foliage which contains an aromatic oil. On an average, the foliage has up to 0.8 percent of oil, containing 60-80 per cent of citronellal that imparts to it the lemon like odour. Commercial plantations exist in the Nilgiri Hills. A plantation is raised on well drained gravelly soils both in tropical plains and in the sub-temperate hills up to about 2000 meters above sea level. Seeds may be sown during early spring either in polythene bags in the nursery or direct in the field. About 10-20 cm tall seedlings are translanted in the field (without exposin their roots) during the rainy season at 45 x 30 cm spacing. The land is usually given 50 kg each of P and K per hectare at planting, supplemented with about 100 kg of N per hectare in 2 to 4 split doses anually as top dressing. The terminal branches are cut to induce the plants to produce more lateral branches. During harvesting, the plants are cropped in April and November and a small harvest is also gathered during the rainy season. Fresh leaves and tender branches are distilled. The average yield from the third year onwards is about 20 tonnes per hectare per annum. This field, in turn, gives about 100 kg. of oil. The price of oil depends upon the content of citronellal in the oil. The Tamil Nadu Cinchona Department has located trees whose foliage is found to possess 85-90 per cent of citronellal and this oil fetches better price.

Muskdana or Ambrette (Abelmoschus Moschatus)

Abelmoschus moschatus (L.) Medic, Malvaceae (Syn. Hibiscus abelmoschus L.) is a tropical weedy shrub native to India valued for its scented seed. Ambrette is a close relative to Okra, a popular horticultural crop. The genus Abelmoschus has six species distributed in the South and South East Asia and in North Australia. Abelmoschus moschatus Medic., A. manihot (L.) Medic., and A. esculentus (L.) Moench, contain wild and cultivated forms, and A. ficulneus, A. crinitus, and A. angulosus, are only wild. Abelmoschus manihot. In Hindi, it is popularly known as mushkdana, kasturi bhendi (kasturi= musk; bhendi= lady's finger). In other Indian languages it is known as gukhia korai (Assamese), kasturi bhenda (Telgu), kattukasturi (Malylam), varttilai kasturi (Tamil), lalkasturika (Sanskrit). The area under ambrette is presently low in India but is increasing rapidly with seed exports to France, Germany, Japan, Singapore, Spain for its use as an aromatic oil. Indian drug manufacturers are introducing new herbal drugs containing ambrette for medicinal use

Botany

Erect hispid herbs or undershrubs, 0.5-2.5 meters high, with a long slender tap root. Leave extremely variable, lower suborbicular in outline, cordate, lower or palmately 3-7 lobed, upper narrower, hastate or sagittate at the base with linear-oblong or triangular lobes. Flowers regular, bisexual, involucral bracts 8-12, hairy yellow with purple centre. Fruits capsule fulvous hairy, oblong lanceolate, acute. Seeds subreniform and blackish.

Uses

Ambrette oil obtained from seeds possess an odor similar to that of musk and its aromatic constitents have long been used in perfumery industry. Different grades of essential, or aromatic absolute, are marked in Europe as high-grade perfumes (Singh et al. 1996) The seeds are valued for the volatile oil present in the seed coat. Seed analysis report 11.1 percent moisture, 31.5 percent crude fiber; 14.5 percent lipids, 13.4 percent starch, 2.3 percent protein, volatile oil (0.2-0.6 percent) and ca/ 5 percent resin.

Analysis of volatiles report myricetin-3-glucoside and a glycoside of cyanidin in flowers, an aromatic constituent in seeds, beta-sitosteral and its beta-D-glucoside, myricetin and its glucoside in leaves and petals and beta-sitosterol from dry fruit husk. In India, roots, leaves (rarely), and seeds of ambrette are considered valuable traditional medicines. The bitter, sweet, acrid, aromatic seeds are used as a tonic and are considered "cooling, aphrodisiac, opthalmic, cardiotonic, digestive, stomachic, constipating, carminative, pectoral, diuretic, stimulant, antispasmodic, deodorant, and effective against "kapha" and "vata," intestinal complaints, stomatitis; and diseases of the heart, allays thirst and checks vomiting. According to Unani system of medicine seeds allay thirst, cure stomatitis, dyspepsia, urinary discharge, gonorrhea, leucoderma and itch. Roots and leaves are cures for gonorrhea . Even use against venomous reptiles has been reported.

Cultivation

Ambrette is cultivated as pre-kharif crop in India. It is usually sown in March–April but as late as the first week of July in Central India. Seed rates of 41g/kg are optimum. Application of dried Neem leaves (500Kg/ha) at last ploughing increased oil content and quality. April sown crop start flowering in September; fruits ripen from November to January and are harvested when fully mature. Applications of fertilizers improves growth of plant and seed yields but studies conducted by SOPAM indicate the use of chemical inputs resulted in negative impact on oil content and quality. Harvested capsules are sun dried and seeds dehisce when the capsules burst. The oil for perfumery is extracted by steam distillation of crushed seeds.

3

Indian Systems of Medicine Plants

"India suffers today in the estimation of the world, more through the world's ignorance of her achievements than in the absence or insignificance of these achievements", observes by IGIEC. This statement is well borne out in the case of ancient Indian medicine. The achievements of Indians in the field of medicine are but imperfectly known to the world even today. The ancient Indian medical classics, written exclusively in Sanskrit, were not easily accessible to any but Sanskrit scholars. Even in India, only a few were acquainted with these classics. The knowledge of medicine was held as a close preserve in a few families of hereditary physicians (*Vaidyas*). These *Vaidyas* were not used to modern ways of thinking, and the idea that they should share their knowledge with others or write books on the subject in other languages to make it known to the world at large, did not appeal to them.

In the early days of Sanskrit studies, the European scholars concentrated their attention mainly on philology and general literature. It was only much later that their studies were directed to the earlier and more important literature of the *Vedas*; but even then these studies did not extend to the medical classics. The commencement of the 20th century witnessed the publication of 'The Encyclopedia of Indo-Aryan Research'. This monumental work, covering the whole domain of Indo-Aryan antiquity, contained many valuable studies on ancient medicine. The colossal task of translating into English the *Charaka Samhita* was successfully accomplished by Kaviratna Avinash Chander. The *Susruta Samhita* was translated into English by Kaviraj Kunja Lal Bhishagratna. These translations have made the great Indian medical classics easily accessible to the English-speaking world. The discovery of the Indus Valley Civilization has considerably widened the horizon of Indian medicine, and has pushed its antiquity back to about 2500 B. C., thus making this civilization contemporaneous with the three non-Aryan civilizations of the ancient world.

ORIGIN OF ANCIENT INDIAN MEDICINE

Ayurveda

Ayurveda is the name which the ancient Indians gave to their science of medicine. *Ayuh* means life and *veda* to know or attain. Ayurveda is the science by the knowledge of which life can be prolonged or its nature understood. The Vedas are the earliest sacred books of India. They are four in number, viz., *Rigveda, Samveda, Yajurveda* and *Atharva-veda*.

There was no Veda called Ayurveda. Its existence is a myth. Susruta calls it an *upanga* of the Atharvaveda. It was raised to the status of a Veda and appended to the Atharva-veda to give the science of medicine the necessary sanctity and authority. There are two versions of its origin. The medical school traces its origin to *Bharadvaja*, who received it from the god *Indra*. The surgical school traces its origin to *Dhanvantari* who received it also from this god.

The universe, according to ancient Indian thought, is composed of five basic elements, the *Pancha Mahabhootas*, namely: Prithvi (earth), Apya (water), Teja (fire), Vayu (air) and Akash (ether). Ayurveda believes in the theory of *Tridosha*: *Vata, Pitta* and *Kapha*. Vata is a combination of two elements of the universe, namely air and ether, Pitta an amalgam of fire and earth and Kapha the combination of ether and water. According to this theory, the Tridoshas remain in a balanced state in the human body in a healthy state and their disequilibrium causes disease.

Health according to Ayurveda, is the natural state of all the three aspects of human being i.e. body, mind and the soul in complete harmony. When the natural state comes in contact with unhappiness, disease results. According to Ayurveda, true medicine is one which cures the disease without causing any side effect. Ayurveda enjoys an advantage over the modern system of medicine. Ayurvedic practitioners take into consideration the body constitution of a patient before prescribing any medicine. They study the state of the body fluids, blood, flesh, fat, bone marrow, semen and vital essence. A regulated diet is prescribed along with the medicine. The regimen of diet is as important as the medicine since former helps restore the balance as much as the latter.

Siddha

Siddha medicine, was originated around 5000 BC in southern parts of India. The word *Siddha* means "an object to be attained", "perfection" or heavenly bliss". According to this system, human body is composed of 96 *Tatwas*, 72, 000 blood vessels and 1300 nerves. Besides these, there are 10 *Nadi* (main arteries), 10 *Vayu* (vital pranas) and 10 *Vegangal* (natural functions). All of them play important roles in different functions of the body.

The Siddha medicine also recognises the role of three humors, called *Mukkuttram* (Vatam, Pittam and Kapham). These humors remain in a balanced state in a normal healthy person and disturbance in their equilibrium leads to ill health. *Siddha* physicians base their diagnosis on Mukkuttram and Ennvagai Thervu.

Yoga

Yoga is a method by which one can develop one's inherent powers in a balanced manner. It offers the means to reach complete self-realisation. The literal meaning of the Sanskrit word *yoga* is "yoke". Accordingly, Yoga can be defined as a means for uniting the individual spirit with the universal spirit of God.

Concept and practice of Yoga originated in India several thousand years ago. Its founders were great Saints and Sages. The great *Yogis* gave rational interpretation to their experiences of Yoga and brought about a practical and scientifically sound method within everyone's reach. Yoga today is no longer restricted to hermits, saints, sages, it has taken its place in our everyday life and has aroused a worldwide awakening and acceptance in the last few decades. The science of Yoga and its techniques have now been reoriented to suit modern sociological needs and lifestyle. Experts of various branches of medicine including modern medical science are realising the role of these techniques in the prevention of disease, mitigation and cure of disease and promotion of health. Yoga is one among the six systems of Vedic philosophy. Maharishi Patanjali, rightly called the "Father of Yoga" compiled and refined various aspects of Yoga systematically in his "Yoga Sutras". He advocated the eight-fold path of Yoga,; popularly known as "Ashtanga Yoga" for all-round development of human personality. They are-*Yama, Niyama, Asana, Pranayama, Pratyahara, Dharana, Dhyana and Samadhi*. These components advocate restraint observance of austerity, physical postures, breathing exercises, restraining the sense organs, contemplation, meditation and *samadhi*. These steps are believed to have a potential for the improvement of physical health by encouraging better circulation of oxygenated blood in the body, retraining the sense organs and thereby inducing tranquility and serenity of mind. The practice of Yoga prevents psychosomatic disorders/diseases and improves an individual's resistance and ability to endure stressful situations.

Unani

The Unani system of medicine owes, as its name suggests, its origin to Greece. It was the Greek philosopher-physician Hippocrates (460-377 BC) who freed medicine from the realm of superstition and gave it the status of science. The theoretical framework of Unani medicine is based on the teachings of

Hippocrates. After Hippocrates, a number of other Greek scholars enriched the system considerably. Of them Galen (131-210 AD) stands out as the one who stabilised its foundation, on which Arab and Persian physicians like Rhazes (850-925 AD) and Avicenna (980-1037 AD) constructed an imposing edifice.

In India, Unani system of medicine was introduced by the Arabs, and soon it took firm roots in the soil. The Delhi Sultans, the Khiljis, the Tughlaqs and the Mughal Emperors provided state patronage to the scholars and even enrolled some as state employees and court physicians. The system found immediate favour with the masses and soon spread all over the country.

According to the principles and philosophy of Unani Medicine, disease is a natural process, its symptoms are the reactions of the body to the disease, and the chief function of the physician is to aid the natural forces of the body. Unani medicine is basically based on Humoral Theory.

Homoeopathy

Homoeopathy is a system of therapeutics based on the Law of Similars as expressed by maxim "Similia Similibus Curentur"-let likes be cured by likes. Dr. Christian Friedrich Samuel Hahnemann is the father of Homoeopathy. In India, this has been recognised as one of the National Systems of Medicine. Homoeopathy came to India as early as 1810 when a French traveller Dr. Honigberger who learnt Homoeopathy from Dr. Samuel Hahnemann, visited India. It is a very popular and widely accepted system in India.

Government's assistance

The Indian systems of medicine viz., Ayurveda, Siddha, Unani and Homoeopathy predominantly use plant-based raw materials in most of their preparations and formulations in addition to some materials of minerals, metals and animal origin. The efficacy of these systems thus mainly depends upon the use of pure and genuine raw materials in the manufacture of drugs of these systems. In all, about 1100 medicinal plants are estimated to find their use in Indian Systems of Medicine & Hemoeopathy and 500 out of these are more commonly used in preparation of ISM and Homeopathy drugs.

Forests have been the source of herbs and medicinal plants. In the last few decades, due to the pressure of increasing population, the area under forests has been decreasing and the demand for herbs and plants has been increasing. Therefore, the forest resources are under double squeeze and are not able to meet the full requirement of medicinal plants and herbs.

In order to meet the above situation, the Ministry of Health and Family Welfare had recently organised regional seminars on medicinal plants. These seminars brought together a wide range of experts. These regional seminars were followed by a few workshops organised in various States. On the basis of recommendations of regional seminars and workshops, 45 medicinal plants were finalised. These medicinal plants were considered important for development on priority as they were already on the verge of extinction. The Ministry has been increasing the cultivation of these plants through its Central Sector Scheme. Many of these species like 'Vatsnabh', 'Guggulu', Saqmonia', 'Yastimadhu', etc. are at present imported at a very high cost resulting in an increase in the cost of the prepared drug, sometimes making these drugs out of reach for many.

National Institutes are set up by Department of Indian Systems of Medicine & Homoeopathy for producing graduates and post-graduates for high quality, conducting research and to provide quality medical care. These are: National Institute of Ayurveda, Jaipur, National Institute of Unani Medicine, Bangalore, National Institute of Homoeopathy, Calcutta, National Institute of Naturopathy, Pune, Morarji Desai National Institute of Yoga, New Delhi, National Institute of Siddha, Chennai and Rashtriya Ayurveda Vidyapeeth, New Delhi.

MEDICINAL PLANTS

India is endowed with a rich wealth of medicinal plants. These plants have made a good contribution to the development of ancient Indian materia medica. One of the earliest treatises on Indian medicine, the Charak Samhita(1000 B. C), records the use of over 340 drugs of vegetable origin. Most of these continue to be gathered from wild plants to meet the demand of the medical profession. Thus, despite the rich heritage of knowledge on the use of plant drugs, little attention had been paid to grow them as field crops in the country till the latter part of the nineteenth century.

During the past seven or eight decades, there has been a rapid extension of the allopathic system of medical treatment in India. It generated a commercial demand for pharmacopoeial drugs and products in the country, Thus efforts were made to introduce many of these drug plants into Indian agriculture, and studies on the cultivation practices were undertaken for those plant which were found suitable and remunerative for commerical cultivation. In general, agronomic practices for growing poppy, isabgol, senna, cinchona, ipecac, belladonna, ergot and a few others have been developed and there is now localized cultivation of these medicinal plants commercially. The average annual foreign trade in crude drugs and their phytochemicals is between 60 and 80 million rupees and this accounts for a little over 0. 5 per cent of the world trade in these commodities.

The curative properties of drugs are due to the presence of complex chemical substances of varied composition (present as secondary plant metabolites) in one or more parts of these plants. These plant metabolites in one, according to their composition, are grouped as alkaloids, glycosides, corticosteroids, essential oils, etc. The alkaloids form the largest group, which includes morphine and codein (poppy), strychnine and brucine (nux vomica), quinine (cinchona), ergotamine(ergot), hypocyamine, (beeladona), scolapomine(datura), emetine(ipecac), cocaine(coco), ephedrine(ephedra), reserpine(Rauwolfia), caffeine(tea dust), aconitine(aconite), vascine(vasaca). santonin(Aremisia), lobelin(Lobelia) and a large number of others. Glycosides form another important group represented by digoxin(foxglove), stropanthin(strophanthus), glycyrrhizin(liquorice), barbolin (aloe), sennocides (senna), etc. Corticosteroids have come into prominence recently and diosgenin(Dioscorea), solasodin(Solanum sp.), etc. now command a large world demand. Some essential oils such as those of valerian *kutch* and peppermint also possess medicating properties and are used in pharmaceutical industry. However, it should be stated in all fairness that our knowledge of the genetic and physiological make-up of most of the medicinal plants is poor and we know still less about the biosynthetic pathways leading to the formation of active constituents for which these crops are valued.

During the last two decades, the pharmaceutical industry has made massive investments on pharmacological, clinical and chemical researches all over the world in an effort to discover and still more potent plant drugs; in fact, a few new drug plant have successfully passed the tests of commercial screening. However, benefits of this labour would reach the masses when the corresponding support for agricultural studies for commercial cultivation is provided. Infact, agricultural studies on medicinal plants, by its very nature, demand an equally large investment and higher priority. India, in particular, has a big scope for the development of the pharmaceutical and phytochemical industry.

The Indian Pharmacopoeia (1966) recognizes eighty five drug plants whose ingredients are used in various pharmaceutical preparations. We shall, however, confine our treatment to a few important commercially grown medicinal plants whose cultivation deserves priority in out national economy.

CINCHONA (cinchona ledgeriana Linn. and allied spp.). Sixty-five species distributed in the Andes at elevations of 800 to 2, 800 m, occur mainly in Peru, Bolivia, Columbia and Ecuador. Commercial supplies of the bank are obtained from C. ledgeriana, c. officinalis, C. calisaya, C. succirubra and their numerous hybrids. The cinchona bark yields quinine which is used as a treatment against malaria. Quinine salts are now increasingly used in soft drinks as bittters and quinidine sulphate is use in the treatment of heart troubles, such as auricular fibrillation and venticular trachycardia. Cinchona plantations cover about 1, 600 ha in the Nilgiris and the Annamalais Hills (Tamil Nadu). India, Indonesia and Zaire (the Congo) are major suppliers of quinine products to the world market; the Indian export of quinine salts earns about Rs 10 million annually.

C. ledgerianna Moens is a small tree grown at elevations between 1, 000 and 1, 900 m, mainly in West Bengal. The average total alkaloid content in the root, stem and branch (of plants 10-12 years old) is 7. 21, 6. 01 and 4. 0 per cent of which the quinine content is 5, 4 and 1. 98 per cent respectively. Under less favourable conditions, a hybrid (ledgerianna X succirubra) is preferred; the hybrid has a lower quinine content, but it produces a more robust tree, growth. C. officinalie Linn. is a weak straggling tree, about 6m high. It grows at altitudes ranging from 2, 000-2, 600 m mainly in the Nilgris. The root, stem and branch contain 1. 75-4. 16, 2. 56-4. 42 and 1. 44-2. 35 per cent of quinine respectively. A hybrid, called robusta (officinalisX succirubra) is a hardy type and, as such, is adapted to a wider range of elevations (1, 2000-3, 000 m) and temperatures; another hybrid (officinalisX ledgeriana) is grown in Mungpoo (Darjeeling District).

C. calisaya Wedd. is a large tree which is not suitable for growing under excessive cold and humid conditions, is grown at lower altitudes of 400 to 1, 000 m in the Moyar Valley (Nilgiris). The total alkaloids in the stem bark range from 3. 89 to 7. 24 per cent, of which quinine and cinchonidine are 0. 78 to 5. 57 and 0. 03 to 1. 56 per cent respectively.

C. succirubra Pavon is a hardy tree which grows between elevations of 1, 200 and 2, 000 m in some parts of Annamalais and attain a heught of 18-20 meters. This species possess a remarkable ability to withstand both high humidity and drought. Its main alkaloid is cinchonidine. The total Alkolid in the root, stem and bark is 7. 6, 5. 5 and 3. 3 per cent respectively. Out of these amounts, quinine constitutes 0. 76-1. 42, 1. 1-1. 74 and 0. 8-1. 76 per cent respectively in the root, stem and bark. Cinchona prefers deep, well drained rich loamy to clayey loam, acidic soils (pH 4. 5-6) on sloping sheltered locations. Most species prefer high humidity, a well-distributed rainfall of about 150 cms, and only minor variation in the maximum and minimum temperatures during their growing seasons. All species are susceptible to frost and succumb to water-logged conditions.

Cinchona is usually propagated through seeds. The seeds are small and light (350-400 seeds per gramme) and loose viability soon. About 50g of fresh seeds sown per square meter during February-May produce about 10, 000 seedlings in the nursery-beds, prepared with a mixture of leaf-mould and sand.

The nursery is provided with partial shade and kept moist and free from weeds. Germination takes 25 to 40 days to be completed and the seedlings grow 4 pairs of leaves in 4 to 6 months when they are transplanted in another nursery at 10 cm X 10 cm spacing. The seedling grow 30-50 cm high in the next 4 to 5 months and are planted in the field at a spacing of 2 m x 2m; the young-growing plants are provided with shade. The plantation is thinned when 4 to 6 years old and thus about 50 per cent of the stock is uprooted and debarked in two years. More bark is obtained in the 8th year by coppicing when only one strong stump is allowed to grow. The left-over trees are finally uprooted when 12-years old. The bark is moved by ringing the stem at a height of 60 cm from the ground and is dried in the open. The drying reduces its weight to 60-70 per cent.

In Indonesia, the vegetable propagation of selected clones has helped to maintain a high quinine content, thereby upgrading the average quinine content from 4 to 7. 5 per cent. Several methods of vegetative propagation, as patch and slit-budding, cincturing, layering and mould-layering, are recommended. Vegetative propagation is done during the monsoon, when root initials are produced in 40 to 60 days and the shoot is then cut off and planted.

The cinchona bark has 30 chemically related alkaloids, of which quinine ($C_{20}H_{24}O_2N_2$) is the most important. The alkaloids are formed during the descent of the sap and, therefore, its percentage is lowest in the twigs and it rises in the stem and is maximum in the root bark; the collar portion of about 30-45 cm in length is the richest portion. The percentage of total alkaloids increases till the age of 8 to 12 years and then begins to decline.

Damping-off is reported both from nursery and fields, particularly at lower elevations. The disease is controlled by fumigation with chloropicrin. Root-rot due to Fomeslamayensis (Murr.) Sacc. and Trott. has also been reported in nurseries; a better drainage of the nursery-beds and spraying with Bordeaux mixture help to prevent it.

ISABGOL (plantago ovata Forks.). It is an annual stemless herb, a native of Persia, now grows as a cash crop on about 16, 000 ha in the Mehsana, Palampur and Banaskantha districts of Northern Gujrat, India is the largest producer of isabgol and exports seed and huskworth Rs 25 million annually. The husk is the rosey-white membranous covering of the seed which constitutes the drug and is given as a safe laxative, particularly beneficial in habitual constipation, chronic diarrhoea and dysentery.

Isabogal is an irrigated rabi crop which remains in the field for about 4 months. The crop is grown in marginal, light, well-drained sandy-loam to loamy soils having pH between 7 to 8. It requires a cool climate and dry sunny weather or light showers cause seed shedding.

After harvesting the kharif crops, e.g. jowar (Sorghum vulgare), the land is brougt to fine tilth and laid out into beds of convenient size for irrigation.

It is preferable to mix with the soil 15 cartloads of well-rotted farmyard mannure per hectare during the preparation of the land. The optimum sowing time is early November; sowing however, is extended till the end of December, but the delayed sowing decreases the yield. The seed rate is 7. 8 kg per hectare. Seeds are small and light about 6000 to a gramme and are sown by broadcast. They are covered thinly by raking the soil. A light irrigation is given immediately. Germination starts in 6 to 10 days and the crop is given the second irrigation after 3 weeks and a third one at the time of the formation of the spikes; thus the crop needs 6 to 7 irrigations.

Isabgol makes a moderate demand for nutrients. Usually, 25 kg of each N and P per hectare is given at plantation. The crop is given 1 or 2 hand-weedings during the entire growing period. The plants are about 50 cm high andeach plants gives out between 25 to 100 tillers, depending upon the fertility of soil and weather conditions. The plant bears the flowering spikes in about 60 days after sowing and matures in the next 2 months. The yellowing of the lower leaves is an indication of maturity, confirmed by pressing a spike between two figers when the mature seeds come out. The crop is harvested close to the ground in the early morning hours to avoid looses owing to seed shedding. The harvested material is stacked for 1 or 2 days, made to be trampled by bullocks, winnowed, and the separated seed crop is collected. A boldseeded crop fetches a better price.

The seeds are processed through a series of grinding mills to seperate the husk, and about 30 per cent husk by weight is thus recovered. The husk contains a mucilaginous substance.

Powdery mildew sometimes attacks the crop and is brought under control by spraying the crop with wettable sulphur, e.g. 'Karathen' and 'Sulfex' two or three times at 15-day intervals after the appearance of infection. White grubs are reported to damage the roots; soil treatment with 5 per cent Aldrin or Lindane to protect the crop is given at the time of the last ploughing during the preparation of the field.

OPIUM POPPY (papaver somniferum Linn). Poppy is a native of the western Mediterranean region, introduced into India in the early sixteenth century. India produces about 70 per cent of the world's production and 90 per cent of it is exported annually. The crop can be grown under a licence issued by the Excise Department and, as such, its cultivation is restricted to about 24, 000 hectares in the districts of Neemuch, Mandsaur and Ratlam in Madhya Pradesh; in Faizabad, Bara Banki, Bareilly and Shahjahanpur in Uttar Pradesh, and in Chittoor, Jhalawar and Kota in Rajasthan.

Poppy is an annual erect plant, 60-120 cm in height, rarely branching, with ovate-oblong leaves; it bears large showy flowers and nearly globose to spherical capsules, containing small white or black kidney-shaped seeds. It is a rabi crop, and remains for about 150-160 days in the fields. It is mainly (90%) self-pollinated, since the dehiscence of anthers takes place before the opening of the flower. A large number of the forms of variety album DC. are cultivated in India; it has ovate globose capsules devoid of apertures.

The crop is grown on well-drained, fertile, clayey loam to rich sandy-loam soils. It prefers moderately cool weather and open sunny locations; severely cold spells, frost dull cloudy weather, high winds, and heavy rainfall during the lancing period adversely affect the yield.

Land is prepared to a fine tilth up to a depth of 20-25 cm during September and the fields are laid out into beds of convenient size. Twenty-five to thirty-seven cartloads of farmyard manure is mixed with the soil during the preparation of the land, penning of sheep or goats is preferred. Seed-rate is 2. 5 to 3. 5 kg per hectare. The seeds are minute weighing 0. 25 to 3. 5 kg per 100. They are mixed with sand and sown thinly in rows 0.3m apart during mid-October till early November (optimum temperature 9-10 degree centigrade). The rows are covered with a thin layer of soil and are given a light irrigation, followed by another irrigation after 8-10 days when the seeds start germinating. Seed treatment with 1.0 % Agrosan protects it from seed-borne dieases. The crop is given about 15 irrigations in all, depending upon the texture of the soil and the variety sown; moisture defiency at the time of capsule formation affects the yield adversely. The crop needs a heavy nutrient supply and 50 kg N/ha is applied during the preparation of the land and another application of an equal quantity is given as top-dressing in two-split doses when the crop is one month old and at the time of the flag-leaf stage. The seedlings are thinned out to 20-25 cm apart when they grow 5-7 cm tall. The crop is weeded and hoed weekly till the plants are about 20 cm tall and thereafter, weeding and hoeing are done once a month. The plants take 75-80 days (in Neemuch, Madhya Pradesh) and about 105 days(in Uttar Pradesh) to come into flower, depending upon the variety sown. The petals fall in 3-4 days and the growing capsule is ready for lancing in the next 6 to 10 days. The green unripe capsules contain the maximum amount of morphine which diminishes with its ripening and yellowing; conversely, codeine and narcotine increases with age.

Lancing is done longitudinally in bright sunlight and the latex (crude opium) which oozes from the wounds dries during the following night and is scrapped with a sharp kitchen-knife in the early hours of the succeeding morning. Lancing is performed in the afternoon with a special knife, capable of making four incisions at a time, each at about 1/12 cm apart. Each capsule is lanced for 4 to 6 times. A deep incision causes the collection of the latex inside the capsule and spoils the seeds. The crude opium is stored in earthen-pots and dried in the sun to obtain the raw opium of a uniform consistency. The dry produce should be stored in closed vessels. The entire produce goes to the Excise And Narcotics Department which pays according to its cosistency and purity. The average yield of raw opium varies from 13 to 33 kg per hectare, though much higher yields are recorded under good agronomic practices. The crop also yield 3 to 4 quintals of seeds per hectare. The seeds contain up to 50 per cent of a golden-yellow fatty oil which is devoid of narcotic properties.

There are 25 opium alkaloids identified in the raw opium. Of them, morphine, theabine, codeine, narcotine and papaverine are important; morphine is by far the most important. The Indian produce of raw opium contains, on an average, about 20% of the total alkaloids by weight. They, in turn, posses 9 to 14% of morphine, 5-7% narcotine, 1. 25-3. 75% codeine, 0. 4-1% papverine and 0. 2-0. 5% theabine. The produce obtained in Turkey and the Balkan countries is collected from one incision only and is therefore rich (10-21%) in morphine; conversely, the Indian opium is richer in codeine and narcotine.

The crop is attacked by the leaf-miner (phyllocnistis sp.), which can be kept under control by spraying with 0. 2% Metasystox or Rogor. Sometimes, cutworms {Agrotis suffura Hubn.) cause damage to the young plants; the flooding of the fields makes these worms float on the water and they are ultimately pickedby birds. Downy mildew (Peronospora arborescens (Berk) de Bary) sometimes causes serious damage to the crops at the time of capsule formation. It is controlled by the application of 0. 2% Diathane Z-78. Root-rot due to Rhizoctonia is also reported on the crop.

SENNA (Cassia angustifolia Vahl.). Sena is a native of South Arabia and is now naturalized in the Tirunelvelly and Ramnathapuram districts of Tamil Nadu. India is the main producer of this crop in the world and exports senna leaves and pods worth over RS 6 million annually. The leaves and the pod-shell contain the laxative principle (sennocide) which is extensively used as a laxative in medicine.

The crop is grown on marginal red lateritic soils. The growing areas of (Tirunevelly and Ramnathpuram) have no distinct winter season; the average maximum temperature (november to February) is 18.3c and the region is received in autumn from the northeasterly monsoon.

Senna is a small, perennial, branched undershrub, remaining in field for 5 to 7 months. It is grown as a pure crop as well as a mixed crop with gram, gingelly, chilles and cotton. Generally, two sowing seasons are recognised, i.e. February to March (irrigated crop) and November (rainfed crop). The seed-rate is 27 kg per hectare under rainfed conditions and 15 kg per hectare for the irrigated crop. The seeds are broadcast or preferably drilled in lines, 30 cm apart. As soon as the seedlings emerge one to two hoeings are given and the plants close up the rows as they grow. This crop genetrally gets the benefit of residual fertiliser applied to the preceding paddy crop and, therefore, in actual practice it is seldom given fertiliser. The application of 20 kg of N and 40 kg of P per hectare at planting, supplimented with 40 to 60 kg/ha of N in 3 split doses is perferred.

The crop is given 5 to 8 irrigations when grown on garden soils. It flowers in about 2 months after sowing and the first flush of flowering stalks is removed to induce a higher degree of branching. The picking of leaves starts in early May and the leaves are stripped off by hand when fully grown, thick and bluish; the second picking is taken alogwith the plucking of pods. The pods are harvested a little before maturity to maintain their green colour; the second crop of pods is obtained at the end of the season when the plants are uprooted during August or April-May. The leaves and the pods are dried in a thin layer in shade for 4 to 7 days; the pods are lightly beaten during drying to remove the inter seed material.

The careless drying of the harvested crop spoils the colour and lowers its active content. The produce is graded, pressed and finally packed in hessian under pressure for long distance transport. The crop yields 1 to 1. 4 tonnes of leaves and about 1. 5 quintals (about one quintal under rain-fed conditions) of pods per hectare. The produce should contain about 2. 5 per cent of active principles, calculated as anthoquinones. Damping-off is common in the seedling stage. To control the disease, seed treatment with fungicides, e.g. Captain, is recommended. The pods are attacked by a borer during storage, leading to considerable damage.

BELLADONNA (Alropa belladonna Linn) It is European species, presently grown on a small scale in Kashmir. Thc plant is a small perennial herb which grows up to 1. 5 m in height. It branched freely and produces a large tapering root. The leaves and roots of belladonna constitute the commercial drug which contains atropine, hyocyamine and hyocine, used in pharmacy for their mydriatic, analgesic and antispasmodic properties; the roots are used for external application only. The leaves and roots should contain not less than 0. 3 and 0. 4 percent of the total alkaloids calculated as hyocyamine. A. acuminata Royel is a closely related Indian species, found at altitudes between 1800 and 3000 meters in the western Himalayas; its leaves and roots contain similar alkaloids. A part of belladonna alkaloids and their products used in India are imported.

The crop prefers a well-drained slightly acidic, siltyloam to clayey-loam soil, rich in lumus. It cannot stand water-logged conditions. It is a crop of the temperate climate, prefers a sunny location and clear whether, particularly preceding and during the harvesting of the crop; continuous dampness or high humidity favours root-rot.

The crop shows a wide variation in growth and alkaloid content in its plants population. Seeds from selected plants with high alkaloid contents should be used for raising a plantation. Propagation through seed is the easiest and least expensive method, through vegetative methods, such as shoot, root and root-shoot cuttings are also used. The seeds are very small, weighing about 700 per g. They should be treated with ethyl alcohol for 3 minutes or with petroleum either for 6 minutes for improving germination. The treated seeds should be washed in running water for a few hours to remove the adhering chemicals. The seeds are sown in rows in the nursery during early spring. Germination takes place 10 to 21 days and is 15 to 40 per cent. Therefore 4 kg of seed gives enough seedlings to plants in one hectare. The seedling bearing 1 to 3 leaves are planted in the field during august at 45 x 60 cm. or 60 x 60 cm. spacing. Ridge planting is preferred in localities receiving heavy monsoon rains. The land is given about 40 tonnes of farm yard manure, besides 100 kg. of diammonium phosphat and 30 g. of K_2O per hectare before planting and 20 kg. of N is given at the time of branching and each time the crop is picked. The plantation is given to 2 to 3 weedings and hoeings before the first leaf crop is obtained and then I or 2 hoeings are usually given before each leaf picking.

The crop is irrigated after every 10 to 15 days during summer. The first picking of leaves is obtained in October; in subsequent years, 3 to 4 leaf crop are obtained for the next three years. Harvesting is done by cutting the plants 20 to 25 cm. on bright sunny days above he ground, except at he time of the autumn harvest when the plants are cut 3 cm. above the ground. The stumps put forth fresh growth during the succeeding spring and bear flowers during June-august and the berries are produced in October. The alkaloids are synthesized in the root and are translocated through the stem to the leaves.

The harvested crop is dried rapidly in the sun for 2-3 days and the leaf-stalks are detached only after the produce is dried. The plants are unrotted after three or four years; the thicker are sliced into 3-4 cm. long pieces and dried. The crop loses 70-80 per cent of its weight during drying. A well dried leaf crop retains its green colour. The average crop yield in the first year is 300 kg. of leaves and thereafter, 750 kg. of leaves per hectare annually. An additional root crop of 2-3 quintals per hectare is obtained when the plants are finally uprooted. Hire average yields of 1-1. 2 tonnes per hectare are reported from European countries. The produce should be stored in cool dry place away from light.

Cutworms (AGROTIS flammatra) attack the tender growing seedling during yearly summer. The application of 5 percent ahe Aldrin dust at 20-25 grammes per square meter of the nursery-bed before sowing protects the crop. The beds may be dranched with 1 : 19 wettable solutions of chlordane, 2-3 times after every 10 days during the attack of the pace. Sometimes damping off of seedlings is caused by pythium sp. and chloropicrin is recommended as a fumigant. Root-rot also damages the crop; the affected plants along with the adhering soil are removed and burnt. Seeds treated with the Agrosan generally protect the seedlings from soil-borne diseases.

RAUWOLFIA (Rouwolfia serpentina Benth) It is an evergreen, perennial indigenous herb found widely distributed in the Himalayan foothills and Peninsular India. The root constitutes the drug and its virtues as an important medicine, were known to the ancient Ayurvedic physicians; it contains 55 alkaloids, reserpine being the most important. The root powder or other preperations containing its alkaloids are prescribed in the treatment of high blood pressure, insomnia, and certain forms of insanity. Roots of rauwolfia and its products command a sizeable market both in India and abroad.

Rauwolfia grows in sandy-loam to clayey-loam acidic soils, rich in humus. It prefers tropical to subtropical climate, receiving heavy monsoon rains between June and August, and the temperatures between 10 and 38 degree centigrades are considered ideal for its growth. The plants sheds its leaves during winter under conditions obtaining in northern India.

It is a one-and-a-half to 2 year crop and can be grown from seeds, root, root-shoot and shoot-cuttings. The seed-crop, however, gives larger (root) yields. The seed rate is 8 to 10 kg per hectare, the average germination being only about 15%. Heavy seeds are selected by floating them in water. They are placed under a moist piece of cloth for 24 hours to soften their hard covering they are sown in well prepared seedbeds in lines, 20cm apart, during April May. The germination is erratic and takes 3 to 8 weeks; the seedlings grow 5 to 8 cm. tall in the next 2 months and are transplanted in well-prepared field at spacing of 45 * 35 cm, 45 * 45 cm, 45*45cm, 45*60 cm or 60*60 cm, depending upon the fertility of the soil and on the intercrops proposed to be grown. The seedlings generally do well and gaps, if any, are filled by fresh planting. The land is preferably mannered with 45 tonnes of farmyard manure per hectare. The crop is given 90 kg of N; 45 kg of p_2o_5 and 45 kg of k_2o per hectare in all; half of n and the entire quantity of superphosphate and potash is given as basal dose and the remaining N is preferably applied in two split doses, one 75 days after planting and the other during the succeeding spring.

The crop is given monthly irrigation from January to May and after a period of 40-45 days during autumn. Rauwolfia has a deep root-system and is a drought-enduring species; continuous drought, however, reduces its total yield. The crop requires 5 weedings and hoeings during its entire growing period. Whereas a heavy root crop is obtained when rauwolfia is raised as a pure crop, the growing of intercrops, such as maize, cowpea or brinjal, during kharif and radish, wheat or a cole crop, during rabi, gives larger overall profit. The roots are dug-out from November (in northern India) to January February in (southern India). The root bark the thin fibrous roots contain a larger percentage of alkaloids and should not be damaged a loss during digging. The roots are dried in the sun, and 55-60 percent of their weight is lost. The average yield is 950 kg. per hectare.

Adults of Anomalapolita feed on the leaves of rauwolfia during the rainy season and are controlled by spraying 0. 2 percent folidol. Sometimes, mosaic also affects the young growing leaves and inflorescenc. Nematode infestation is restricted to acidic soils. A wilt due to Fusarium sp. and leaf-blight due to Alternaria sp. and reported to cause minor damage. Sometimes a brown leaf spot is found on the lower surface of the leaves caused by Cercospora rauwolfiae. Die-back is caused by Colletotri-chumdematium, particularly under humid growing conditions. The affected branched may be pruned and the plants are sprayed with 0. 2 percent Diathane Z-78 which controls the spread of the disease.

IPECAC (Cephaelis ipecacuanha (Brot.) A. Rich, It is a perennial, evergreen, straggling herb, upto 50 centimetre tall, inhabiting the tropical forest of the south America. It produces slender 10-30 cm. long and 4-10 cm. thick, annulated crockery rhizones. The root bark is the drug of the commerce, used as an expectorant and emetic, mainly in the treatment of amoebic dysentery. The measure world supllies come from Brazil and the neighbouring countries. India, however, is one of the few countries which grow this crop commercially; its cultivation is done by the West Bengal Cinchona department in the Darjeeling district and to a smaller extent in Sikkim and parts of Assam. The annual production ranges between 25 and 30 tonnes of dry roots and part of the produce, including emetine salts, is exported earning a foreign exchange of 1 million rupees annually.

The crop prefers warm and moist sandy loam forest soil, rich in humus and potash. A high well distributed rail fall (minimum 200 cm.), a temperature range of 10 to 38 degree centigrade and the altitudes of 500 to 600 meters, and sides shelter from strong wind constitute the most suitable environment for ipecac cultivation. The crop could be raised from seeds shoot and root cuttings. The vegetative propagation, however, shortens commercial varieties are known, mainly after the name of the country of origin. Seeds are small and are sown by broad cast by during January and March in well prepared and heavily manuared raised seedbeds of convenient size. About 35 g. of seed is sown per square meter.

The average germination is 30 percent and the seed take 3-5 months to germinate. The seedbeds are shaded during the day and kept moist and free from weeds. Seedlings about 4 cm. tall, are transferred to the rooted nursery, with 5x5 cm spacing between the plants after the monsoon rains are over. They remain there till the following March and April, when they are again transferred to a third side with spacing of 20x20 cm. between the plants. The plants remain there for three year till the roots are dug out.

Ipecac is thus slow growing 4 year crop which is very exacting in its requirement for continues shad, moist beds (but no water logging) and regular interculture. The plants give out dark green elliptical leaves and bear white flowers and small dark-purple globose berries in the second year. The flowers are dimorphic, heterostylous (and therefore cross pollinated) and are formed in group of 6-8. The berries ripen during September-October. The seed is white, plano-convex, 5-6 x 1. 5-2 mm. and is cover with a hard tests. About 1/3 of the seeds are sterile. The growing plants require a good amount of nutrient supply which is mainly added to the soil through heavy organic manuring; information on the use of inorganic fertilizers is not known. Each plant forms 2-3 long rhizomes which are dug out during dry weather; the rhizomes are cleaned of the adhering soil and rapidly dried in the direct sun for 2-3 days. The dry rhizomes are broken into smaller pieces and finally packed in bales for transporting to the extraction sides. The yield varies from 600-1000 kg. of roots per hectare.

The roots contain emetine caphaeline and psychotrine as its main alkaloids; emetine, however is the most important. The average total alkaloid content in the Indian crop is 2. 5 percent of which 1. 3-1. 4 percent is emetine. The alkaloids are extracted in the form of their salts viz. emetine sulphate and emetime hydrocloride, for marketing. According to the Indian pharmacopoeia (1966), the ipecac, of which not less than 50% should consist of nonphenolic alkaloids.

The seed beds are sometimes infested with Fusarium and rhizoctonia spp. causing damage to the plant suitable fungicids may be used to control the infection of the plants.

FOXGLOVE (Digitals lanata Enrh). An exotic biennial herb, cultivated mainly in central and southern Europe for leaves which contain glycosides used for heart stimulation. India imports a major parts of its requirements of this drugs. The crop perfers silty-loam to clayey-loam soils, rich in organic matter and temperate climate (1200-2000 m above the sea-level). The seed-rate used is 500 grammes per hectare. The nursery is raised in early spring and seedlings, when 8-10 weeks old, are transplanted, 30x45 cm to 60x60 cm apart, depending upon the soil fertility. It is an irrigated crop and makes only a moderate demand for nutrients, mainly as nitrogenous and phosphatic fertilzers. The plants flower in the second year, but the flowering stalks are removed to induce a larger leafy growth. In general, one harvest of the leaf crop is obtained in October in the first year, whereas 3 harvests of leaf crop are obtained in the second year. The average yield recorded in India in the second year is 600 kg/hs; higher yield up to 1, 500 kg are reported from elsewhere. Digitalis leaves are thermolabile and hygroscopic and therefore, should be rapidly dried at 40 C immediately after collection. They should contain 0. 1% glycoside (digoxin, digitoxin, gitoxin, etc.) calculated as lanatocide-c and not more than 5% moisture. The leaves could be stored in the form of coarse powder in airtight containers placed in a cool and a dry place.

DILL OR SOWA (Anethum graveolens Linn.). Sowa is a rabi crop grown almost throughout the country for its fresh aromatic leaves used in cooking, and its fruits are marketed as a common condiment.

The fruits contain an essential oil, rich in carvone and is used in pharmacy for the preparation of dill water and similar preperations to treat flatulence, abdominal and colic pain. India exports dill fruits worth about Rs 2 million annually. There are two known varieties, viz. the East Indian Dill (A. graveolens var. sowa) and European Dill (A. graveolens Linn.); the former alone is cultivated in India commercially; its oil possesses superior aroma, but is considered inferior in pharmacy owing to the presence of a toxic substance (dillapiole) which is, however, easily removed.

Dill prefers well-drained fertile loamy soil and can be raised under a wide range of climatic conditions. The seeds are sown direct in the fields in rows or along the bunds in early autumn and the seedlings are thinned after about 40 days of sowing to maintain a spacing of 60 x30 cm. The crop is given 40kg each of N, P and K per ha at planting and another 40kg of N as top-dressing, depending upon the fertility status of the field. The crop mature by the end of April in northern India and green mature umbnles are picked in 10-25 days to avoid seed-shattering. The average yield comes to 1 tonne of fruits per ha. The sowa seeds on distillation yield 2. 5 to 3 per cent of an essential oil rich in arvone which imparts to the oil its characteristic flavour.

Powdery mildew (Erysiphe umbelliferum forma anethi) sometimes causes heavy damage to the crop and is controlled by 2 to 3 sprayings of sulphur at 25 kg/ha during the early flowering stage. Aphids occasionally cause damage; the spraying of Malathion (0. 5%) 2 to 3 times during infection is recommended.

LIQUORICE OR MULHATI (Glycyrrhiza glabra Linn.). Liquorice is a hardy perennial legume, about 0. 6 m tall, found wild in countries of west

Asia. Its dried peeled or unpeeled underground stems and roots constitute the drug. It is demucent, mildlu laxative, expectorant and, as such, is an important constituent of all cough and catarrh syrups, throat lozenges and pastilles; its extract containing glycyrrhizin (2. 14%) has a healing effect on peptic ulcers. Large quantities of liquorice root is used in confectionery and tobacco-blending. There are a number of commercial cultivation varieties of liquorice, such as typical Regal and Herd. (Spanish liquorice) which is the sweetest of all and therefore, fetches higher price; var. glandulifera Waldst and Kit. (Russian liquorice) is richer in glycyrrhizin but the sweet taste is accompanied with perceptible but mild, bitterness owing to the presence of liquiritin and isoliquritin; var. violaca Boiss. (Persian liquorice) produces thich, hard and lumpy roots and is considered inferior in quality.

Liquorice grows well in fertile sandy-loamy soils in a warm and dry climate, having a long growing season marked with well-defined winters to induce the translocation of food to the underground perennating rhizomes. Heavy rain or frost affects its growth adversely. Most of the growing areas fall around 14N latitude. The crop is raised from rooted cuttings which are planted in early spring 90 x 60 cm apart in rows. The beds are worked up to a depth of 1 metre and liberally mannered. Seeds are seldom used. Var. typically produces a strong taproot which gives out rhizomes, whereas var. glandulifera sends out rhizomes are ready for harvesting in 3 to 4 years and are dug out in autumn after rains. A portion of the harvested material is decorticated before drying to produce the peeled liquorice of commerce. The material is cut into pieces, 15-20 cm long and 1 to 2 cm in diameter, and are dried alternatelly in shade and the sun. This drying reduces the weight of the material to 50 per cent. Artificial drying can also be done at 30-40 C. The crop yield ranges from 1 to 3 tonnes per hectare, depending upon the soil fertility, the variety, the climate and cultivation practices.

DIOSCOREA. The tubers of a number of non-edible dioecious species of Diocorea provide raw material for the industrial production of corticosteroids is around 300 tonnes, valued at about Rs 3, 000 million. Of the several species, D. composita Hemsl, and D. floribunda Mart. and Gal. (from Central America) and D. deltoidea Wall. ex Kunth. (from western Himalayas) and D. prazeri Prain and Burk. (from Eastern Himalayas) stand out prominently because of the higher percentage of diogenin content in their tubers. Of late, a D. floribunda clone, developed at the Indian Institute of Horticultural Research, Bangalore, has been found to grow fast and give exploitable tuber yield in about 18 months of the growing period.

The crop of Discorea floribunda is raised from tuber pieces, each weighing 50-70 grammes, treated with a stemic fungicide for protection against soft-rot; these tuber pieces are planted in pits at 60 x45 cm spacing during March-April. The tubers sprout between 30 and 60 days after planting. Each pit is given 1.5kg of farmyard manure or compost along with 30 kg each of N and P per ha at planting, supplemented with similar quantities of fertilizers during the rainy season. Another application of 60 kg of N+40kg of P is given in 2 split doses in the second year. The growing vines are given support for getting the optimum uy\yield. The tubers grow up to 30 cm depth in the soil and, being soft, should be dug out carefully. An average yield of 1 kg of fresh turbers, containing 70 per cent moisture, per plant is reported from Bangalore. The calculated tuber yield as reported, is 7. 5 tonnes (dry) per ha, containing, on an average, 3 per cent diogenin.

MEDICINAL PLANTS - A HUGE FAMILY

Medicinal plants as a group comprise approximately 8000 species and account for around 50 per cent of all the higher flowering plant species of India. There are estimated to be over 7800 manufacturing units in India. The Indian Systems of Medicine have identified around 1500 medicinal plants, of which 500 species are mostly used in the preparation of drugs. The medicinal plants contribute to cater 80 per cent of the raw materials used in the preparation of drugs. The effectiveness of these drugs mainly depends upon the proper use and sustained availability of genuine raw materials.

Around 70% of the medicinal plants in the country are spread across the tropical forests of the Western ghats, the Vindhyas, the Nagpur plateaus, Aravalli, the Terai region and the wide areas of the Himalayas and the North East. The diverse climatic conditions of India is suitable for cultivation and especially medicinal plants which has helped in finding of the Indian Systems of Medicine (ISM) which is slowly developing into a form of alternate medicines globally.

The domestic market of Indian Systems of Medicine & Homoeopathy is of the order of Rs. 4000 crores per annum, which is expanding day by day. The Ayurveda drug market alone is of the order of Rs. 3500 crores. Besides this, there is also a growing demand for natural products including items of medicinal value/pharmaceuticals, food supplements and cosmetics in both domestic and international markets.

According to the statistics released by DGCIS at the end of the year 2003, India's total export earnings from the sale of crude drugs and herbal extracts, stood at around Rs. 512 crores per annum. On adding the export earning from "finished products" the export figure went up by another Rs. 222 crores to reach a total of Rs. 734 crores per annum. At the beginning of 2003, if we take into account the average annual rate of growth of Indian exports during the previous years (15%) India's export turnover is probably of the order of Rs. 971 crores.

It is estimated that the export earnings would be raised to Rs. 3000 crores annually by 2005.

India, with its diversified biodiversity has a tremendous potential and advantage in this emerging area. In recent years, the growing demand for herbal product has led to a quantum jump in volume of plant materials traded within and across the countries. An estimate of the EXIM Bank puts the international trade in medicinal plants at US $ 60 billion per year and growing at the rate of 7 per cent.

Research and Development

Medicinal plants are used at household and institutional level in a self-help mode. One and a half million practitioners of ISM & H use medicinal plants in preventive/promotive and curative applications. There are about 4, 60, 000 registered practitioners of ISM&H using medicinal plants in the codified streams. Pharmacies are mostly owned by family companies and most of them are secretive in trade and largely unregulated.

At present, 90% collection of medicinal plants is from the wild, generating about four million man days employment (both part and full time) and since 70% of plants collection involve destructive harvesting many plants are endangered of vulnerable or threatened. Similarly, the medicinal plants are collected without paying attention to the stage of maturity. They are stored haphazardly for long period of time under unsuitable conditions. This results in deterioration of quality. Despite the wealth of resources (biological, human and financial) available, the sector has not developed in the absence of suitable standardization, quality control, efficacy of drugs.

In order to fully convert the potential of our medicinal plants into economic wealth, a very active Research and Development (R&D) programme is essential. The R&D has to cover all aspects relating to the species from collection to utilization. For convenience we may categorize medicinal species into:

Those which are of proven medicinal value as per scientific parameters;

Those on which sufficient leads are available; and

Those on which further investigation and examination are required to be done.

It is desirable to have a 'need based' approach to research on medicinal plants including screening of plants for biological activity. Research efforts could thus be directed for a number of above-mentioned diseases for which suitable drugs are not available in the modern system of medicine and where herbal drugs have a possibility of offering new drugs. Focused R&D, inter

– disciplinary approach research is the crux of accelerated development of this sector.

The search for new drugs of plant origin has yielded fruitful results in the past. In terms of a modern research endeavour, drug development from plants must necessarily imply a multi-disciplinary approach. It is necessary to prioritize the thrust areas to obtain the output of research efforts and other resources.

Several factors help in determining the priorities. These include the distribution of flora, national or regional disease pattern, availability of modern health care etc. In addition we have to keep in mind the global priorities in developing new drugs so as to get a good financial return.

In the wake of all these developments, the governments of various nations are being challenged to develop appropriate policies to regulate the use of such traditional medicinal products. At present, the policies of the developed countries are not favourable for freely trading in traditional medical products.

For the reason that most of the traditional medical products that are introduced into the market are not backed up by rigorous scientific studies to establish their safety, efficacy and standards, they are not recognized as drugs. On the basis of a preliminary documentation of their use in traditional medical systems in the country of origin, selected products are being certified as diet or nutritional supplements.

There is a need to enforce strict regulations for Good Agricultural Practices (GAP), Good Laboratory Practices (GLP), Good Manufacturing Practices and Good Clinical Practices (GLP).

It is a long-felt need of the herbal industry and traditional medicine sector in India to emerge as a strong forum under one umbrella to partake in the growing global market for herbal and traditional medicine.

After initial consultations with all the stakeholders, the Federation of Indian Herbal Industry (FIHI) have been launched on 28 February 2004 at Chennai.

It is expected that FIHI will streamline and strengthen the partnership between Government, industry and the scientific community and to protect, project and promote traditional healthcare systems and products. This will act as a link between the growers, industry, research institutions and the consumers.

Holistic Approach to Healthcare

In India, as in most other countries, traditional and modern medical systems have always co-existed. Today patients make their decisions depending on their culture, perceptions and assessment of either system's capacity to solve their health problem, as also on the accessibility and affordability of the healthcare systems.

The ideal situation is an integrated holistic medical service system, which assimilates the valuable knowledge of different systems so that the patients benefit optimally.

It is the duty of not only the Government and the NGOs, but also the medical service industry to see that there exists an integrated holistic healthcare system so as to offer the best care for the patient.

This conference will focus on the relevant issues of Health Insurance, Patents and legal issues at the role of farmers in terms of growing medicinal plants. There is a huge business potential in this sector, which amounts to more than US $100 billion per annum. We need to promote this service sector in the international market.

It is therefore evident that Allopathic, Herbal and Complementary Healthcare Practitioners and Professionals, Health Insurance Providers, Hospitals including Rural Health Centers and all sections of Academia should engage in a dialogue to contribute to this common goal.

MEDICINAL PLANTS : THE GLOBAL VIEW

Human beings have been utilizing plants for basic preventive and curative health care since time immemorial. Recent estimates suggest that over 9, 000 plants have known medicinal applications in various cultures and countries, and this is without having conducted comprehensive research amongst several indigenous and other communities.

Medicinal plants are used at the household level by women taking care of their families, at the village level by medicine men or tribal shamans, and by the practitioners of classical traditional systems of medicine such as Ayurveda, Chinese medicine, or the Japanese Kampo system. According to the World Health Organization, over 80% of the world's population, or 4. 3 billion people, rely upon such traditional plant-based systems of medicine to provide them with primary health care.

Allopathic medicine too owes a tremendous debt to medicinal plants: one in four prescriptions filled in a country like the United States are either a synthesized form of or derived from plant materials. Even from the earliest trade data available, it is clear that the global market for medicinal plants has always been very large.

According to the International Trade Centre, as far back as 1967, the total value of imports of starting materials of plant origin for the pharmaceutical and cosmetics industry was of the order of USD 52. 9 million. From this amount, the total values grew to USD 71. 2 million in 1971, and then showed a steady annual growth rate of approximately 5-7% through to the mid-1980s. To give an example of the extent of trade volumes even at that time, according to one report commissioned by the World Wide Fund for Nature, the total import in 1980 of "vegetable materials used in pharmacy" by the European Economic Community was 80, 738 tons (Lewington 1992). India was the largest supplier by far, with 10, 055 tons of plants and 14 tons of vegetable alkaloids and their derivatives.

However, it is only during the last decade that the real significance of the medicinal plants sector has begun to be realized. Interest in natural materials by the dominant economic powers had waned from the late 1960s to the early 1980s as new possibilities in biotechnology and the synthesization of drugs beckoned. But by the mid-1980s, there was a renewed interest in natural materials and approaches to health care, coupled with a recognition that technology alone could not solve the pressing health care needs of the world's population (Tempesta and King 1994).

This new drive for natural and plant-based medicines made itself felt in the market from the mid-1980s onwards. Growth in the market in various regions is now on average 3 to 4 times the average growth rates of the national economies in the same regions. Some of these phenomenal rates, in some cases nearly 20%, imply that the market is now doubling in size every 4-5 years. The participation of various companies in the market also attests to its new strength and importance. By 1990, some 223 major companies worldwide (of which about half were in the United States) were reportedly screening plants for new leads; the figure had been zero in 1980 (Aryal 1993).

Also in 1990, more than 2000 companies in Europe alone were marketing herbal medicinals, with 30% having a turnover in excess of $20 million-expenditure in the United States on "unconventional, alternative, or unorthodox" therapies reached $13. 7 billion dollars during the same year (Tewari 1996).

The so-called "nutraceuticals" sector—consisting of herbal medicines which are dubbed food or dietary supplements in order to pass FDA criteria more easily—is now estimated to be valued at USD 27 billion (Anon 1995).

Table : Natural Medicines Market: Regional Growth Rates 1991-98 (in %)

Region	1991-92	1993-98
EU	5	8
Rest of Europe	8	12
SE Asia	12	12
Japan	15	15
South Asia	15	15

The use of such alternative medicines has become increasingly popular in the developed world. For example, 1 in 3 Americans have at some time used unconventional medical therapies according to a national telephone survey published in the New England Journal of Medicine in 1993. In another survey conducted in 1994, it was found that 60% of doctors had at some time referred patients to practitioners of alternative medicine. In response to the overwhelming interest in alternative therapies, many of the prestigious allopathic medical institutions have also recognized their importance: an example is the National Institute of Health which created the Office of Alternative Medicine in 1991 to provide the public with information on alternative treatments and to assess those therapies which have proven successful. According to one account, in 1992 significant amounts of at least 74 species of medicinal plants were being commercially traded in the global market (Handa 1992). In addition to these major species, hundreds of others are bought and sold in lesser quantities across national boundaries, sometimes illegally.

A comparison of the volumes of traded materials with those of the previous decade also provides dramatic evidence of the market's growth. During the last 3 years, approximately 40, 000 tons of plant drug materials (valued at DM 160 million) were imported into Germany, annually (Lange 1996), implying that one country's imports in the mid 1990s equalled half the number of plants imported by the entire continent in the mid 1980s.

CHALLENGES IN MEDICINAL PLANTS SECTOR

The continuous increase in human population is one of the causes for concern in meeting the daily requirements of food and medicine as the economy and livelihoods of human societies living in developing countries primarily depend on forest products. This phenomenon is leading to continuous erosion of forest and the forest products, thus making challenge to meet the requirements as well as to conserve useful bio-resources. More and more species are being gradually added in the Materia Medica; however, the standards of their purity and correct identification do not keep pace with the process of expansion. The market prices for medicinal plants and derived materials provide only a limited insight into the workings of the market, and not on the precise information of profits, supply and demand. We have identified the following major features and challenges on the basis of examining the existing knowledge on the medicinal plants sector.

Rising demand

The World Health Organization (WHO) has estimated the present demand for medicinal plants is approximately US $14 billion per year. The demand for medicinal plant-based raw materials is growing at the rate of 15 to 25% annually, and according to an estimate of WHO, the demand for medicinal plants is likely to increase more than US $5 trillion in 2050. In India, the medicinal plant-related trade is estimated to be approximately US $1 billion per year. According to an estimate, the quantity of export of Ayurvedic products produced in India has tripled between last two financial years (2001–2002 and 2002–2003).

The projected escalating demand of medicinal plants has led to the over-harvesting of many plants from wild, which subsequently results in the loss of their existing populations. For example, the large quantity of Himalayan yew (*Taxus baccata*) has been gathered from the wild since its extract, taxol, was established as a use in the treatment of ovarian cancer. *Aconitum heterophyllum, Nardostachys grandiflora, Dactylorhiza hatagirea, Polygonatum verticillatum, Gloriosa superba, Arnebia benthamii* and *Megacarpoea polyandra* are other examples of north Indian medicinal plant species which have been overexploited for therapeutic uses and have subsequently been placed today in rare and endangered categories. Many medicinal plant species are used in curing more than one disease, and as a result, these species are under pressure due to over collection from wild. For example, *Hemidesmus indicus* is used to cure 34 types of diseases; *Aegle marmelos* 31, *Phyllanthus emblica* 29, and *Gloriosa superba* 28. Over-exploitation and continuous depletion of medicinal plants have not only affected their supply and loss of genetic diversity, but have seriously affected the livelihoods of indigenous people living in the forest margins.

More than 95% of the 400 plant species used in preparing medicine by various industries are harvested from wild populations in India. Harvesting medicinal plants for commercial use, coupled with the destructive harvest of underground parts of slow reproducing, slow growing and habitat-specific species, are the crucial factors in meeting the goal of sustainability. Harvesting shoots and leaves of medicinal plants may decline their photosynthetic capacity, and as well as the potential for survival and effective propagation. Medicinal plants tolerance to harvest varies with climatic conditions as the temperate herbs become highly vulnerable to harvest of individuals. Furthermore, rising demand with shrinking habitats may lead to the local extinction of many medicinal plant species.

Increasing rarity

The continuous exploitation of several medicinal plant species from the wild and substantial loss of their habitats during past 15 years have resulted in population decline of many high value medicinal plant species over the years. The primary threats to medicinal plants are those that affect any kind of biodiversity used by humans. The weakening of customary laws, which have regulated the use of natural resources, are among the causes of threatening the medicinal plant species. These customary laws have often proved to be easily diluted by modern socio-economic forces. There are many other potential causes of rarity in medicinal plant species, such as habitat specificity, narrow range of distribution, land use disturbances, introduction of non-natives, habitat alteration, climatic changes, heavy livestock grazing, explosion of human population, fragmentation and degradation of population, population bottleneck, and genetic drift. Additionally, natural enemies (i.e., pathogens, herbivores, and seed predators) could substantially limit the abundance of rare medicinal plant species in any given area.

In addition to the consumption of medicinal plants by animals, there are physical ailments in humans, which are cured by different species of the same genera. For example, the malarial fever is treated by many species of *Swertia* (e.g. *Swertia chiraiyta, S. angustifolia,* and *S. cordata*). Similarly, different species of *Berberis* (e.g. *Berberis aristata, B. asiatica, B. lycium, B. chitria* and *B. jaeschkeana*) are used as a source of berberidine to cure certain eye diseases.

Furthermore, different species of the same genera contain different proportions of chemical quantity, and there is a preference over their demand; however, the degree of threat for their exploitation is relatively lower than those species, which do not have alternatives

An estimated 4,000 to 10,000 species of medicinal plants face potential local, national, regional or global extinction, with subsequent serious consequences for livelihoods, economies and health care systems. Although, a few studies exist on the rare and endangered medicinal plant species of the northern India, none of these studies have complete data set for even a single species. In 2003, 71 rare and endangered medicinal plant species have been assessed for the northwest Himalaya during the Conservation Assessment and Management Plan workshop, according to the guidelines of the World Conservation Union. In northern India, *Aconitum* is the rarest genus with 5 species, followed by *Rheum* with 4 rare species. Out of the 71 rare medicinal plants, 92% are in active trade; 74% are traded nationally and 35% are traded internationally.

The meager availability of data on the population and quantum of rare species in nature, however, has restricted their categorization to a few species on the basis of herbarium collection and by consultation by a few experts. The present assessments are also questioned for their validity on the assignment of threat categories to the species, including the number of taxa in danger for specific area. The problems in assessing the species is increased in the mountainous region, especially high altitude areas because of tough and inaccessibility of the terrain, inhospitable climatic conditions, and short life cycle of plants. Most of the available data have been collected from the easily accessible areas in these mountains. Indigenous communities and commercial herb gatherers also raid these same areas for collection of medicinal plants. Therefore, the estimated population density of categorized rare medicinal plants is not precise because it differs the areas that never and hardly undergone any collection of such rare medicinal plant species.

CULTIVATION OF MEDICINAL PLANTS

Information on the propagation of medicinal plants is available for less than 10% and agro-technology is available only for 1% of the total known plants globally. This trend shows that developing agro-technology should be one of the thrust areas for research. Furthermore, in order to meet the escalating demand of medicinal plants, farming of these plant species is imperative. Apart from meeting the present demand, farming may conserve the wild genetic diversity of medicinal plants. Farming permits the production of uniform material, from which standardized products can be consistently obtained. Cultivation also permits better species identification, improved quality control, and increased prospects for genetic improvements. Selection of planting material for large-scale farming is also an important task. The planting material therefore should be of good quality, rich in active ingredients, pest-and disease-resistant and environmental tolerant. For the large scale farming, one has to find out whether monoculture is the right way to cultivate all medicinal plants or one has to promote polyculture model for better production of medicinal plants.

Studies conducted on the agro-forestry of medicinal plants elsewhere suggest that since many medicinal plant species prefer to grow under forest cover, agroforestry offers a convenient strategy for their cultivation as well as conservation through: 1) integrating shade tolerant medicinal plants as lower strata species in multistrata system, 2) cultivating short cycle medicinal plants as intercrops in existing stands of tree crops, 3) growing medicinal tree as shade providers and boundary markers, and 4) inter-planting medicinal plants with food crops.

Notwithstanding, it is understood that the cultivation of medicinal plants is not an easy task as the history of medicinal plants farming reflects. Many farmers in trans-Himalayan region of northern India have replaced the medicinal plants farming with common crops [i.e., peas (*Pisum sativum*), potatos (*Solanum tuberosum*) and hops (*Humulus lupulus*)] due to the lengthy cultivation cycle of medicinal plants like *Saussurea costus*. The cost of many medicinal plants in northern India is lower than many seasonal vegetables, which is a cause of scanty farming of medicinal plants.

Attempts are being made by different organizations to cultivate various medicinal plant species, including rare and endangered categories. Agro-technology for about 20 species of rare and endangered medicinal plants of the northern India has been developed by different organizations. However, the per hectare cost of cultivation, total annual production and cost benefit ratio fluctuate with different medicinal plant species. Out of 10 selected rare and endangered medicinal plant species, *Rheum emodi* was calculated as a most beneficial cash crop of the medicinal plant in terms of net income generation in northern India. At present, however, the farming of most of the medicinal plant species is being operated on a small scale and is restricted to a few hectares of land in various states of northern India. There is an uncertainty of obtaining the necessary permits from government agencies for cultivation of medicinal plants. Additionally, many farmers are unaware about the agency responsible for issuing permits. If the farmers are not granted permits needed to cultivate, they are forced to sell their products on the illegal market, which exposes them to action by government agencies and the exploitation by middlemen.

BIO-PROSPECTING AND BIO-PIRACY

The former remote green forests have now become part of a dynamic, profit-seeking economy and demanding pluralistic politics worldwide. Reducing the pressure on various forest products, especially on the medicinal plants, is therefore a tough challenge both for policy makers and for economists. Medicinal plants are the local heritage with global importance. The Convention on Biological Diversity at Rio had agreed on a framework that would help the biodiversity to be utilized in a prudent and controlled way. Bio-prospecting, at present, occurs in an environment of suspicions and growing tensions between the bio-piracy and rights of sharing benefits between the developing and developed countries. Most of the issues relating to the protection of the legal status for indigenous knowledge and compensation of the indigenous herbal practitioners for that knowledge are extremely complicated. There are arguments for the present state of compensation or benefit sharing under the intellectual property rights, which is being considered a new legal form of bio-piracy by one group, whereas other groups argue that the intellectual property right is a legal tool to protect the rights of knowledge holders.

Different ways and systems for awarding patents on the medicinal plants in India, United States, Europe, Canada and other countries have widened the confusion. In many countries, the plants and inventions directed to the plants and the plant products (i.e., seeds, flowers, gums, and resins) are not eligible for filing a patent. In United States, however, any living organism derived by human invention, such as by breeding or by laboratory-based manipulation, can be filed for awarding patent. The Indian Protection of Plant Varieties and Farmers Rights Act of 2001 recognizes the contribution of farmers who actively participate in the breeding programs. Furthermore, this act contains provisions for benefit sharing whereby local communities are acknowledged as a contributor of plants.

Unfortunately, there is a wide gap between developed and developing nations such as India on patenting the products. For example, out of the 3,125,603 patents filed in 91 countries, only 301,177 or 9.6% are registered in developing countries while the rest is in industrialized countries. Of these, only 0.2% of the total and 2.3% of those registered in developing countries belong to residents. In addition, 97.7% of the total patents filed thus far are in the name of non-residents, who apply solely to control export markets in developing countries. Developing nations and many scientists who want to exploit medicinal plants demand more specific rules about the recording of nationality of samples and sharing of their benefits between the nations of origin, the inventor, and the commercial sponsors. Some developed nations are not inclined to accept such provisions. These conflicts have frustrated many scientists who believe that natural products remain the most promising source for new drugs. To mitigate such conflicts and gear up to find out new sources for drugs, the representatives of 188 nations at Kuala Lumpur Conference in 2004 agreed to try to build such a framework that would be acceptable to all signatories and thus the proposed framework will be placed for consideration at the next meeting in 2006 going to be held in Brazil.

Strengthening legalized market system

Besides government agencies, there are numbers of stakeholders ranging from herb gatherers, local middlemen, urban traders, wholesalers, manufacturers, exporters and herbal healers in the medicinal plants trade sector. The marketing system in medicinal plants sector is largely unregulated and inequitable. The medicinal plant collectors are generally the marginal farmers and laborers.

They get cash income to meet their basic requirements for food, health and children education by selling medicinal plants. They are often unaware about the real market prices of many medicinal plant species. Generally, in medicinal plants sector, there is a top down approach and even the many stakeholders at the bottom are not aware of the rising demand of their product and the availability of its market. In some villages of Chamoli district of Uttaranchal, the farmers had cultivated Kut (*Saussurea costus*) and Dolu (*Rheum emodi*) but they were unable to sell them due to lack of knowledge on the marketing system. Conversely, many medicinal plant species are traded through illegal channels.

The other constraints in the medicinal plants sector are: 1) slow rate of production of many medicinal plants, 2) long gestation period, 3) shortage of suitable cultivation technology, 4) production of small quantity, 5) unscientific harvesting, 6) paucity of research on the high yielding varieties, 7) inefficient processing techniques, 8) fluctuation in demand and supply, 9) poor quality control procedures, 10) scarcity of good manufacturers, (11) poor marketing infrastructure, and 12) poor coordination among different stakeholders. On many occasions, the wild medicinal plants are preferred by manufactures compared to the cultivated ones, as there is a general feeling that wild plant species contain better chemical contents. The variation in chemical contents also depends upon the harvesting seasons of species and different stages of species growth. The medicinal plant sector is largely less documented and inadequately regulated. The economy generated by this sector is therefore, not precise because of the enormous illegal trade. The economic benefits and management cost for wild populations are poorly estimated on several occasions.

OPPORTUNITIES IN DEVELOPING THE MEDICINAL PLANTS SECTOR

For developing the 'herbal industries', the northern India possesses a rich diversity of medicinal plant species across the various forest types along an altitudinal gradient (as discussed in the use and diversity of medicinal plants). Such a high diversity of medicinal plants would be helpful for further scientific research on exploring their medical efficacy, value addition, and use in curing various old and new diseases. India has already established a reputation as a low-cost manufacturer of high quality generic drugs in the global market. This fact can be used as an important tool for the marketing of herbal products produced in India. It is expected that India's aim to build a golden triangle between traditional medicine, modern medicine, and modern science will be a boon for developing the traditional herbal medicine and the medicinal plants sector.

Existing policies

In the National Five Year Plans of India, the medicinal plants sector has been identified as an integral part of the Indian System of Medicine and Homeopathy. In 1983, the National Health Policy recognized that the large stock of health manpower in Ayurveda, Siddha, Unani, Homeopathy and Naturopathy had not been adequately utilized; therefore, steps need to be taken to move towards a meaningful integration of the indigenous and modern systems of medicine. The Planning Commission and the National Medicinal Plants Board (NMPB) of the Government of India have prepared a policy document on the promotional and commercial aspects of the medicinal plants sector. In addition, the NMPB has prioritized 32 and Planning Commission has enlisted 24 medicinal plant species for research and development in order to meet the desired aim of the medicinal plant sector. The Biodiversity Act 2002 has framed many rules for sustainable utilization of medicinal plants and to mitigate the chances of bio-piracy.

According to Uttaranchal state action plan, the Forest Department of the state will have to identify two major areas in each Forest Division; namely the conservation area and the developmental area. The conservation areas will be selected based on their rich medicinal plants diversity and marked for *in-situ* conservation and complete protection in the concerned Forest Division. In the developmental areas, apart from protection of the existing bio-resources, the medicinal plant species of the neighbouring areas will also be introduced and cultivated at a large scale. The remaining areas in the Forest Division will remain open for sustainable harvesting of the medicinal plant species. A Joint Harvesting Team, composed of medicinal plants experts, Forest Department officials and some selected local people, will be constituted, which will decide the extent of annual harvesting of the desired medicinal plant species. The various policies at national and state level and their subsequent implementation will provide an opportunity in the advancement of medicinal plants sector. This model of conservation and cultivation of the medicinal plants may be useful for generating the raw material for the 'Herbal Industries' as well as for ensuring the conservation of the rare medicinal plants.

Institutional support

In India, many government and non-government organizations have had the focused attention on improving the medicinal plants sector. Opportunities for funding have been created to assist the person who is willing to work and to build capacity of the medicinal plants sector. According to the mandate of NMPB, the projects may be submitted for funding within two major schemes: *viz.*, a promotional scheme and a commercial scheme. The major thrust areas within the promotional scheme are: 1) survey and inventory of medicinal plants, 2) *in-situ* conservation and *ex-situ* cultivation of selected medicinal plants, 3) production of quality planting material, 4) diffusion of knowledge through education and communication, 5) promotion of global and domestic market system, and 6) strengthening research, development and man power. Within the commercial scheme, the major thrust areas are: 1) bulk production of medicinal plants and ensuring supply of quality planting material, 2) expansion of selected medicinal plants farming areas, 3) value addition in harvesting, processing and marketing of medicinal plants, and 4) developing innovative marketing mechanism.

Apart from the two major themes, the role of NMPB is to co-ordinate with the different ministries, departments, organizations, state and union territory Governments in order to develop and strengthen the medicinal plant sector. One of the major roles of NMPB is to make contacts with national and international organizations devoted to similar mandates and goals. A total of 35 State Medicinal Plants Boards have also been created by NMPB for the smooth functioning of the medicinal plants sector. Approximately 35,000 hectares of land has been selected and brought under cultivation under the supervision of NMPB for the large-scale farming of commercially important medicinal plants. One of the schemes of NMPB is a contractual farming in which any group, institution or person that possesses at least 3 years of experience in medicinal plants sector would be eligible to receive at least 30% financial assistance of the total project cost.

Ten years before establishment of NMPB (during 1992–93 financial years), a single project was launched to study the medicinal plants of the Himalayan region. During past one decade, there has been a considerable expansion in the Himalayan medicinal plants research as it is evident that many projects have been launched exclusively on the medicinal plants during that period. Of the total 4254 projects sanctioned by NMPB over past 5 years, 732 projects have been sanctioned to 11 hill states in northern India. All these projects are expected to strengthen the medicinal plants sector, to bridge the gaps and to meet the challenges in developing the sector. In addition to major funding organizations, the G.B. Pant Institute of Himalayan Environment and Development has sanctioned projects on the medicinal plants of northern India under the scheme of Ministry of Environment & Forests. The Council of Scientific and Industrial Research is building up a Traditional Knowledge Digital Library, which will contain > 35,000 herbal medical formulations used in Ayurvedic system of medicine.

The National Bank for Agriculture and Rural Development (NABARD) has established a policy with a viewpoint to develop a suitable environment for financial institutions by providing bankable models for some 50 medicinal and aromatic crops with the unit cost and scale of finance at the state level. Additionally, NABARD assists in supporting the capacity building of prospective entrepreneurs through Rural Entrepreneurs Development Programs by providing 100% refinancing. NABARD has also close linkages with the NMPB and different State Medicinal Plants Boards. Attempts have been made by various organizations at different levels to establish and promote the medicinal plants sector.

RECOMMENDATIONS FOR DEVELOPING THE MEDICINAL PLANTS SECTOR

The present worldwide interest in plant-based medicines of Indian origin needs to be harnessed by reframing a clear policy for the promotion of commercial cultivation, research and development, and for the increase in exports of medicinal plants. For the development of the medicinal plant sector, there is a need to develop the coordinated efforts at each stage (e.g. research, cultivation, collection, storage, processing, manufacturing and marketing), which would be supported by an appropriate policy framework. Some problems and their remedies for the medicinal plants-based economic venture.

Selection of medicinal plant species for cultivation is an initial important step for the development of the medicinal plants sector. Economic feasibility is the major rationale for a decision to bring medicinal plant species into cultivation. Apart from the priority species selected by the Planning Commission and the NMPB, the rare species banned for collection from the wild should also be taken on a priority basis for cultivation because a majority of such species are very expensive, have high demand and low supply. Cultivation may not be economical if a medicinal plant species is abundant in the wild and easily collected. Therefore, the less abundant species in the wild should be promoted for the large-scale cultivation. Farming of any medicinal plant species should be brought into practice only after the reliable cultivation technology of the concerned species is available. A large variation in climatic and soil conditions in northern India sustain a variety of medicinal plant species, which may be cultivated according to their niche.

For developing the medicinal plants sector, there is a need to: 1) document indigenous uses of medicinal plants, 2) certify raw material for quality control, 3) develop and improve the agro-technology for valuable medicinal plants, 4) officially recognize and protect the customary laws of indigenous people, 5) prepare a clear policy for granting permits for cultivation within stipulated time, 6) conduct regular research and training on better harvesting and processing techniques, 7) investigate various pathological agents infecting medicinal plants, 8) setup a community-based management of medicinal plants farming and marketing, 9) analyze the market policies, 10) monitor and evaluate the status of medicinal plants with the assistance of local communities, 11) conserve the critical habitats of rare medicinal plant species, and 12) share benefits judiciously arising from local people's knowledge on medicinal plants.

These attempts may reduce dependency on wild resource base, and generate alternative income opportunities for the rural and underprivileged communities.

The medicinal plants sector can be improved if the agricultural support agencies would come forward to help strengthen the medicinal plants growers, and if research institutions would help the plant growers by improving their basic knowledge about cultivation practices. Awareness and interest of farmers, supportive government policies, assured markets, profitable price levels, access to simple and appropriate agro-techniques, and availability of trained manpower are some of the key factors for successful medicinal plants cultivation. The diffusion of any available scientific knowledge on medicinal plants should be made operational by a network structure of communication. Currently there are number of herbs which are used in curing diseases but are not documented in details due to a lack of communication and relatively low frequency of their uses. The traditional uses of low profile and lesser-known medicinal plants should also be documented to disseminate their therapeutic efficacy by preparing well acceptable medicines and also to reduce the pressure on over-exploited species.

Apart from the more than 9992 licensed pharmacies with 717319 registered practitioners of Ayurveda, Siddha, Unani and Homeopathy in India, there are many unregistered herbal practitioners in India who prepare their own traditional herbal formulations for curing different diseases, and the available herbal formulations should be standardized for their efficacy. Such scientifically prepared medicine will place herbal medicine in a proper perspective and help in getting a broad global market. Some people do try to take advantage through the introduction of less effective medicinal plants in the name of well-established high-value medicinal plants. Such attempts must be discouraged. To discourage such malpractices, the certification of raw material should be done for quality control by using the modern tools such as thin layer chromatography and high performance thin layer chromatography. In addition, high performance liquid chromatography (HPLC), volumetric analysis, gas chromatography, column chromatography, and gravimetric determinations may be used for standardization and for quality control. Various factors relating to pathological agents (e.g. bacteria, virus, fungi and nematodes) and infected medicinal plants should be investigated by identifying the various symptoms of diseases such as mildew, rust, necrosis, spots, blight, rot, wilt, galls, curl and canker to produce the healthy farming of medicinal plants.

On many occasions, the collection of planting material, especially of rare and endangered medicinal plant species from natural habitats for various experimental purposes by researchers, also poses a threat on their natural populations in wild. The researchers must be aware on the germination potential, seedlings and rhizomes survival strategies of the desired species collected from wild for scientific experiments. Researchers must plant a similar number of individuals back in nature after completion of research work on the collected species. There is also a communication problem between researchers and farmers. This communication problem limits a researcher's capability to deal with the farmers' problems. Hence, communication links between researchers, extension services of institutions, and farmers should be strengthened.

The majorities of current research programs on the medicinal plants conservation are being shifted from ecosystems to species levels. Although there are protected areas across the Himalaya, most of the protected areas have a focused attention on the preservation of faunal diversity except for a few protected areas such as the Valley of Flowers in North West Himalaya and the Tipi Orchid Sanctuary in North East Himalaya. There is not a single protected area focusing on the conservation of medicinal plants. Thus, there is an urgent need for identification and notification of areas for the conservation of medicinal plants on a priority basis. Most of the documentation and research on indigenous uses of medicinal plants is focused on the human aspect. Animal husbandry is the backbone of economy in a majority of indigenous societies. Maintaining the good health of livestock will benefit these indigenous societies. Since there are many medicinal plant species used in curing the various animal related disorders and diseases, the research work also needs to be done on the uses of medicinal plants for curing livestock diseases.

Being a part of tradition, there are many other social issues attached with medicinal plants sector. The indigenous knowledge on harvesting, storage and usage of medicinal plants built over centuries needs to be taken into account for improving the sector and allocating scare resources among the competing demands. Development of medicinal plants farming, encouragement of traditional herbal use and herbal healers, establishing medicinal plants conservation areas, establishing the Social Capital Trust for herbal healers, establishment of linkages among various stakeholders, etc., are among some of the social issues that need to be honoured and addressed properly. The folklore on several medicinal plants and the formulation developed by using them is well recognized in different ethnic communities living in northern India. These folklores should be brought into laboratory for validation.

Conclusion

The traditional medical systems of northern India such as Ayurveda and Tibetan are part of a time-tested culture and honoured by people still today.

These traditions have successfully set an example of natural resource use in curing many complex diseases for more than 3,000 years. Many advantages of such eco-friendly traditions exist.

The plants used for various therapies are readily available, are easy to transport, and have a relatively long shelf life. The most important advantage of herbal medicine is the minimal side effects, and relatively low cost compared to the synthetic medicines. The success of medicinal plants sector mainly depends on the awareness and interest of the farmers as well as its other stakeholders, supportive government policies, availability of assured markets, profitable price levels, and assess to simple and appropriate agro-techniques. The successful establishments of medicinal plants sector may help in raising rural employment, boost commerce around the world, and contribute to the health of millions.

4

Indian Medicinal Plants

KNOWLEDGE RELATING TO MEDICINAL PLANTS

Mere knowledge is difficult to protect legally, as it is intangible. One kind of protection is by means of asserting an intellectual property right, such as a patent, copyright, or trade secret. In the case of medicinal plants, traditional knowledge relating to these plants does not fall within any of these established categories. On the other hand, the use of technology, including biotechnology, to develop a useful product using this traditional knowledge is generally protected. The issue of bio-piracy in relation to such useful and financially productive knowledge has come into Knowledge relating to medicinal plants prominence as a result of the cases challenging the patent granted on neem and on turmeric.

In the turmeric case, the US Patent and Trademark Office granted a patent on the "use of turmeric in wound healing". India successfully challenged this patent by showing that this use of turmeric was well known and that nothing new had been invented. The documents relating to this traditional knowledge of India were unknown to the US Patent and Trademark Office. When they were brought to the attention of the Office they were considered to be "prior art" and the patent was revoked.

In the case of neem, the patent challenged referred to improving the storage stability of an insecticide containing neem seed extracts. This patent could not be revoked as the patent holder (W. R. Grace & Co.) had improved on existing knowledge. While neem-based insecticides were well known, they did not have the storage-stability claimed in the patent. The patented composition could thus be distinguished from the traditional knowledge.

The cases of turmeric and neem are illustrative of the dilemma facing India in relation to the traditional knowledge of medicinal plants. On the one hand, traditional knowledge is not documented in an easily accessible form so as to be considered "prior art". On the other hand, where traditional knowledge is available as to the property of a particular plant, it can be modified so as to be distinguishable from the original traditional knowledge for legal purposes. The end result is that a particular company may get the sole right to manufacture and sell the active chemical compound derived from a plant, although communities may have used the plant for the same or similar purpose over a long period of time.

To prevent this, the preparation of databases of traditional knowledge is being actively pursued. This would solve the problem of showing traditional knowledge to be "prior art" (the turmeric case). But this does not solve the problem faced in the neem case that of the modification of traditional knowledge. Information as provided by traditional knowledge is often all that is needed to provide the necessary input for research and development by a pharmaceutical company, which may use it to make a product that is legally "new", but is considered to be bio-piracy by the community concerned.

One solution to this would be to have pre-conditions in place for access to the databases. This would take the form of a legal contract between the researcher and the database owner. This contract may necessarily vary from region to region or community to community, but it would nevertheless be based on certain common provisions. For example, the contract would require the researcher to give an undertaking to give credit to the community as the source of the information, to share any future benefits arising out of the use of such knowledge, etc. The contract would be have to be signed by every person accessing the database, irrespective of country or community or reason for access, before he or she is permitted to look at the database.

Apart from the above non-statutory methods of protecting knowledge, the Biological Diversity Bill, 2000 requires prior approval of the National Biodiversity Authority for any foreigner or non-resident Indian who wishes to obtain knowledge associated with any biological resource occurring in India. Its prior approval is also necessary for any person who wishes to apply for any intellectual property right anywhere in the world for an invention based on information on a biological resource obtained from India (except in the case of a patent application, where the approval may be obtained anytime before the sealing of the patent). The Parliamentary Standing Committee that considered this Bill has recommended that a ceiling of 90 days be provided to the Authority for granting its approval.

The Patents (Second Amendment) Bill, 1999 has a limited form of protection for traditional knowledge. It states that an Indian patent may be opposed or revoked if the invention was anticipated having regard to the knowledge, oral or otherwise, available within any local or indigenous community in any country. This would need to be reciprocated by other countries for Indian traditional knowledge to be adequately protected.

India has adopted a combination of methods for the protection of medicinal plants. Wherever a pluralistic legislative framework is adopted, the efficacy of the system depends to a large extent on the amount of friction between the parts. As each legislative proposal has been promoted by a different Governmental Department, it could be difficult for the national interest to be promoted without close co-operation between the different Authorities involved.

CONSIDERING THE ROLE FOR INDIA

The global context briefly sketched above suggests several tremendous opportunities for India, a country unrivaled in terms of diversity of medical systems and practices, in addition to being a major storehouse of biological diversity, with 2 of the 14 megabiodiversity areas of the world located within its borders. The global market would appear to be more receptive than ever to the mounting of a concentrated Indian effort at supplying it with medical materials and know-how. Such an effort would also appear to be increasingly remunerative for the country. India is of course already an active participant in the global medicinal plants market having been for some time the world's largest supplier of raw materials (though an insignificant supplier of finished products) (Patnaik 1994). Of the 74 species accounted for in one of the studies mentioned above, India was known to be exporting 22 and importing 8 (Handa 1992), while the German study quoted earlier, which is now underway, has found India to be Germany's largest trading partner by far (Lange 1996). Moreover, medicinal plants are one of the most important components of the non-wood forest products sector which supplies over 80% of India's net forest annual export earnings.

Despite these promising indications, however, it is unclear whether India is truly exploiting her comparative advantage in the medicinal plants sector and tapping the full potential of an expanding consumer base. In addition, several concerns arise in relation to the current consequences of participation in the market, with regard to the sustainability and equitability of prevailing practices in the sector.

Although only micro-studies are currently available in this regard, most of these indicate that current practices are both unsustainable, as they rapidly deplete the natural supplies of the country's plant base, and inequitable, perpetuating impoverishment for those charged with stewarding and harvesting the resource, while a few profit in dramatic disproportion to their inputs. Negative impacts on local primary health care, as plants become diverted to national and international markets, have also been cited in some cases. To add to all of these negative aspects, the market in India has been shown to be highly inefficient and imperfect.

The need of the hour, then, is to replan India's participation in the expanding global market, in light of the interests of all the stakeholders who are affected and who play a role in this sector. There is a need to collate all the available information regarding medicinal plants development in the country in order to obtain a comprehensive overview which will provide the necessary insight for coordinated and effective action.

Such an overview could form the basis of a renewed development of India's medicinal plants sector, and a strategic exploitation of her comparative advantage in the global market on a sustainable and equitable basis.

ORIGINS AND OBJECTIVES OF THE REVIEW

It was with the intention of providing such a comprehensive overview that the International Development Research Centre and the World Bank's Department of Agriculture and Natural Resources commissioned the authors to conduct a state-of-the-art review of the medicinal plants sector in India.

Medicinal plants, of course, do not presently constitute a sector as typically defined in international development discourse; generally they have been defined as a forestry sub-sector, or less often, as a sub-sector in health care. However, this review takes up medicinal plants as an independent sector for two reasons: 1) to emphasize that none of the various 'homes' to which medicinal plants have been assigned provide a sufficient base of expertise for their sustainable and equitable development; and 2) to provide an organizational framework for the community of researchers and stakeholders, to whom this paper will be circulated, to think through this area of common interest and move forward together.

This review then is a mapping exercise, which tries to identify the who, what, how, where, why and when of medicinal plants development in India, in order to supply a comprehensive understanding and overall picture to researchers, NGOs, health care workers, private companies, conservation and development agencies, policy makers and other interested stakeholders. It is intended to provide a framework and knowledge base, and an initial way forward, for those interested in seeing India exploit her comparative advantage in the global market, both sustainably and equitably.

LIMITS AND CONSTRAINTS FACED

There is no dearth of interest in medicinal plants amongst the Indian research community. As a single example, the IDRC Medicinal Plants Network, a South-Asia focused initiative operating from New Delhi, already maintains an active database of over 900 Indian researchers and development specialists working on medicinal plants projects after only one year of active compilation.

When a call for proposals in the field was issued, over 250 responses were received within the subscribed period, a tremendous number considering that the grants were of the magnitude of only USD 15, 000.

Unfortunately, however, this interest has not resulted in the development of a strong and high-quality knowledge base for the sector. Instead, one finds in a review such as this one several instances where information is either unobtainable or unreliable. Several factors contribute to this situation.

The most important among these is the highly secretive and complex nature of the trade in raw materials. Most experts consulted agreed that the largest part of the trade occurs in the informal sector, and is absent from official statistics and trade catalogues. As previous authors have also found, nearly everyone involved in the medicinal plants trade is very hesitant to divulge information which is essential to a complete understanding —such as prices, supply sources, points of transformation, and transport routes. As a result, despite assiduous efforts, we still cannot claim to have a complete picture of the trade scenario, and have most likely erred in the direction of conservatively estimating the volumes of materials under trade.

Information available regarding the formal sector is also limited. Most data is available only in aggregate form, such as numbers of species being exported or overall value of the trade to India. These statistics unfortunately supply little information about how the market actually works, and may even obscure such vital information to policy makers such as seasonal fluctuations and the like. In addition, in most cases, no explanations are given for how the aggregations were calculated or verified (i.e. dry weights or fresh weights; exchange values in effect; self-reporting by companies or based on registration with governments, etc.). The lack of methodological explanation makes it virtually impossible to compare and synthesize related sets of information; or to understand why two sets of statistics, purporting to cover the same phenomena over the same time period, give differing results.

Moreover, these statistics rely exclusively on market price as an indicator of value, a narrow approach which neglects environmental, cultural, personal, and long-term methods of assigning value. The social context of the market which is extremely important in the medicinal plants sector, involving as it does, a complex market spread across time and space, is there by lost. This constraint is related to a general lack of strategic focus in the bulk of current socio-economic research on medicinal plants in India. The largest group of scientists currently working with medicinal plants appears to be those in the natural sciences—including botanists, taxonomists, and chemists; and the applied sciences such as biotechnology and health care. In most instances where economic or social analysis has been undertaken, it has been by these same scientists, the majority of whom are untrained and unqualified to conduct such research.

While laudable as an attempt to bridge the disciplinary barrier, this has unfortunatelyalso resulted in a generally lower quality of socio-economic analysis related to medicinal plants as against other resources, with analysis tending to oversimplify complex market and policy realities such as the frequently suggested solution: cut out the middleman. In addition, there is a regrettable absence of any 'research community' or peer group working on socio-economic and policy aspects of medicinal plants, such as that which exists with regard to agro-technology, biotechnology, and the like, which would assist in defining higher standards of quality.

ABRUS PRECATORIUS L. (FABACEAE)

Syn : *Abrus minor* and *A. pauciflorus* Desv.

English names: Indian liquorice, Crab's eye.

Sanskrit name: Krishna gunja.

Vernacular names: Asm : Latuwani; **Ben:** Rati, Kunch; **Guj:** Gumchi; **Hin** and **Pun:** Rati; **Kan** : Gurgunn, Gulaganji; **Ori** : Kaincha, Gunja; **Mal:** Kunnikkura; **Tam:** Kunthamani; **Tel:** Gumginja.

Trade names: Rati, Kunch.

Traditional use: *SANTAL:*

(i) grind the roots, make small pills, encase the pills in molasses and eat the same to treat night-blindedness;

(ii) make a plaster by grinding the roots of white-fruited variety and apply the plaster on the painful part of inflammated sections of the gum;

(iii) to treat white-coloured urine they drink a mixture made by grinding roots of the following:

a. white-fruited *A. precatorius,*

b. *Indigofera pulchella,*

c. *Panicum repens* and

d. *Spatholobus roxburghii;*

e. to treat gravel they drink a mixture made of the following:

- roots of *A. precatorius,*
- the refuse of molasses,
- exudation from a sapling of *Diospyros tomentosa,*
- exudation from *Acacia catechu,*
- little saltpeter, and
- pinch of sulphur;
- to treat the variety of childbed complaints (usually caused by

anaemia) characterized by profuse diarrhoea, roots of A. *precatorius* are used in preparing two different varieties of mixtures; the ingredients of the mixtures are given below:

First variety: roots of *A. precatorius, Elaeodendron roxburghii, Coix lachryma-jobi, Piper longum, Ruellia suffruticosa,* white onion, rhizome of *Zingiber officinale;*

Second variety: roots of *A. precatorius, Coix lachryma-jobi, Embelia robusta, Piper longum,* bark of *Casearea tomentosa, Elaeodendron roxburghii, Gmelina arborea, Emblica officinalis,* white onion, leaves of *Ocimum sanctum,* rhizome of *Curcuma angustifolia* and *Zingiber officinale*-all these are ground together, boiled and mixed with the refuse of molasses;

- roots as abortifacient and in paralysis;
- apply leaf-paste with lime-water (2:1) on swelling of glands;
- grind the leaves of white-flowered *A. precatorius,* warm slightly and plaster on the loins to kill pain there;
- grind leaves of A. *precatorius* along with leaves of *Lawsonia alba* and *Tamarindus indica* (1:1:1), add a little salt, boil a little and apply the plaster on the whole body to get relief from muscular pain caused by over-exhaustion;
- make a paste of leaves of *A. precatorius* along with roots of *Carissa carandas* and *Gossypium arboreum,* warm the paste slightly and plaster the same over the whole body of the patient suffering from stealth convulsions;
- leaf-paste in leucoderma;
- seed-paste in skin diseases;
- seeds after some processing as contraceptive. *MUNDA:* Root-paste in gonorrhoea. *ORAON:* dried root-powder as mild purgative.

AGNI PURANA:

(i) husks of *A. precatorius* along with the same of *Vitis vinifera* and the decoction of *Polyalthia longifolia, Moringa pterigosperma, payomuca* and *triphala* (fruits of *Terminalia belerica, Terminalia chebula* and *Emblica officinalis)* destroys all intestinal worms;

(ii) the mixture of powder of *A. precatorius,* marine salt and *pathya* in warm water removes all fevers;

(iii) consumption of the seeds of A. *precatorius* along with the fruits of *Melia azadiracta, Holarrhena antidysenterica* (leaves). *Acorus calamus* (young leaves) and *Glycyrrhiza glabra* (powder of stem) causes vomiting;

(iv) regular drinking of *A. precatorius* along with *Acorus calamus, Gloriosa superba, vasa, nisagada, Zingiber officinalis, Glycyrrhiza glabra* and marine salt daily in the morning enhances memory of young boys;

(v) A. precatorius can enhance the span of a man's life, if it is eaten with

marine salt and some other plants *(Tinospora cordifolia, pathya, citraka,* dried rhizome of *Zingiber officinalis).*

Modern use: *Roots:* emetic and alexiteric; *Decoction of roots* and *leaves:* for cough, cold and colic; *Seeds:* purgative, emetic, tonic, aphrodisiac, used in nervous disorder and cattle poisoning; *Poultice of seeds:* as suppository to bring about abortion; *Paste of seeds:* applied locally in sciatica, stiffness of shoulder joints and in paralysis.

Phytography : Copiously branched climber with slender branches; leaves alternate, pinnately compound with numerous deciduous leaflets; flowers small, in dense racemes on axillary peduncles or short branches; pods 2. 5-3. 7 by 1. 0-1. 25 cm; seeds bright scarlet and black or whitish or black or mixed black and white, large like pea.

Phenology: *Flowering:* August and September; *Fruiting* : January to March (even up to May).

Distribution: Occurring throughout greater parts of India, ascending the outer Himalaya up to 1200 m, occasionally planted in gardens.

Ecology and cultivation: Naturalised in tropical countries.

Chemical contents: *Root* and *Leaf:* glycyrrhizin, isoflavanquinones, abrusquinone A, B & C; leaves taste sweet and roots less so; roots also contain precol, abrol, abrasine and precasine. *Seed:* poisonous, principal constituents being 'abrin'; a fat-splitting enzyme, haemaagglutinin, urease; alkaloid (abrin), a glucoside (abralin) and a small quantity of fatty oil have also been isolated from seed.

Pharmacologically, abrin is considered to be intensely poisonous. Besides abrin, a seed contains hypaphorine, two steroids-one oily and the other crystalline-â-sitosterol, stigmasterol, 5 B-cholanic acid, abricin, abridin, cholesterol, lectins and toxic protcins.

Remark: *Root* is used as an adulterant of the root of *Glycyrrhiza glabra* (Fam. *Fabaceae).*

AEGLE MARMELOS CORR. (RUTACEAE)

Syn: *Feronia pellucida* Roth, *Crataeva religiosa* Ainslie

English names: Wood apple, Bael tree.

Sanskrit names: Bilwa, Shriphal.

Vernacular names: Asm and **Ben:** Bel; **Guj:** Biliva phal, Bil; **Hin** : Shriphal, Bel; **Kan:** Bilwa patre, Bil patre; **Kon** : Belfoll; **Mal:** Vilvam, Koovalam; **Mar:** Bel; **Ori** : Bela; **Pun:** Bil; **Tam:** Vilvam, Vilvamaram; **Tel:** Bilambu, Maredu; **Urd:** Bel.

Trade names: Bel, Shriphal.

Traditional use: *SANTAL:* (a) *leaves* of this plant along with {i} many other plant materials for the treatment of continuous fever; (ii) the molasses and fruits of *Gryllus monostrosus* for the treatment of diseases without premonitory symptoms; {iii} the fruits of *Nigella indica* and black pepper to *treat* a patient of convulsions; (iv) the leaves of *Melia azadirac hta* and the seeds of *Semecarpus ana cardium* to *treat* nausea; (v) the fruits of *Randia dumetorum* and *Nigella indica,* oilcake of *Bassia latifolia,* salt and *Carum ajowan* for treatment of constipation with meteorismus; (vi) the bark of the following plants -*Pterocarpus marsupium, Bauhinia vahlii, Spatholobus roxburghii, Terminalia tomentosa, Dalbergia latifolia* and fried rice for treatment of chronic stomachache and (vii) the bark of *Odina wodier,* salt and *Carum ajowan* to treat watery diarrhoea; (b) *various parts of fruit* for making the following medicines: (i) for curing the patient of cholera, a medicine prepared with the following, is administered: the old fruit of A. *marmelos,* bark of *Melia azadirachta,* the resin of *Shorea robusta* and pulverized kernel of a mango stone; (ii) a sherbet prepared with the ripe fruit of A. *marmelos* and sugar candy is administered to the patient of dysentery; (iii) to treat the complaints of a mother after child-birth, a plaster made of the following is applied: top of the fresh unripe fruit of A. *mermelos,* leaves of *Ocimum sanctum,* little ginger and 84 blac_ peppers; (iv) a patient of puerperal fever is given a liquid drink made with the entire contents scraped out of a ripe fruit of A. *marmelos,* juice of old dried fruits of *Mangifera indica,* two ounces of a kind of red ants and a little salt; (v) a thick mixture, made with twin fruits of A. *marmelos,* melted hail and earth excavated by rats, is smeared on the breasts of a young mother to check the flow of milk when the breasts pain or suppurate; and (c) the bark of old trees of *A. marmelos* and *Melia azadirachta* are used to prepare an antidote for the poison of all kinds of snake bite; *ATHARVAVEDA* : the unripe fruit medicinal, but ripe fruit harmful; *CHARAKA SAMHITA:* the unripe fruit increases the digestive power, but the ripe fruit is difficult to digest; *KURMA PURANA:* (i) regular drinking of fruit juice ensures long span of life and golden colour of the skin; (ii) brushing the teeth with young branch of this plant is beneficial;

MATSYA PURANA : the paste of this plant is a good steriliser for clothings, beds, furniture, coat of armour, ornaments, canopy and fans made of wools and furs; *BRAHMAVAIVARTA PURANA* : consumption of ripe fruits of this plant helps to eliminate the ailment caused by excessive bile, but drinking water immediately after eating the fruit aggravates the bile-disorder; *AGNI PURANA* : (i) this plant is of great medicinal value; (ii) inhaling the oil, obtained from this plant, increases the poetic acumen of the inhaler and enables him to live a long life; (iii) for treatment of gastroenteritis, the patient should drink (a) the water containing the decoction of A. *marmelos, Aconitum heterophyllum* and *Holerrhena antidysenterica,* (b) the fruit juice of A. *marmelos,*

Mangifera indica, Dolicos lablab, Woodfordia fruticosa, shunthi along with buttermilk and molasses; and (iv) it can cure a patient suffering from fever and its associate pains and cough.

UNANI: Ingredient for 'Belgiri'.

HOMOEOPATHY: Destroys phlegm and a *good* remedy in fevers associated with catarrhal symptoms, also good for dropsy, bleeding piles, dysentery, diarrhoea, bowel complaints and is a good laxative.

Modern use: *Fruits:* chiefly used in (i) chronic diarrhoea and dysentery; (ii) as a good laxative, and the sherbet prepared from the pulp is good for bacillary dysentery; *Half-ripe fruit:* astringent, digestive and used in diarrhoea. It is also antidiuretic, anthelmintic, antipyretic, carminative, tonic.

Phytography: Deciduous glabrous tree, up to 8 min height and 1 m in girth, bark shallowly furrowed and corky; leaves alternate, with straight sharp axillary thorns (buds), trifoliate, aromatic; flowers in axillary panicles, greenish white, fragrant; fruit hard-shelled, up to 5 cm in diameter, greyish or yellowish, scented, pulp orange, sweet and gummy; seeds numerous, oblong, compressed, testa mucous.

Phenology: *Flowering:* April-May; *Fruiting:* persistent, ripening by February.

Distribution: Found in the plains and submontane regions of India, wild in the sub-Himalayan tract, often planted.

Ecology and cultivation: Wild; often planted.

Chemical contents: *Bark of root* and *stem:* umbelliferone, other coumarins, â-sitosterol, aurapten, marmin, lupeol, two unidentified alkaloids and two unknown compounds-their proportion varies with the age of the bark; *Stem:* yields a good gum; *Heartwood:* a ferro-quinoline alkaloid, /dictamine, marmasin and â-sitosterol; *Leaves:* ã-sitosterol, aegeline, aegelenine, lupeol; sitosterol, rutin, marmesinin, â-sitosterol, glucoside and essential oil; *Fruits:* psoralen, aegelinol, furanocoumarin, marmelide, â-sitosterol and essential oil; *Ripe fruits:* xanthotoxol, scoparone, scopoletin, umbelliforone, marmesin, skimmin and â-sitosterol glucoside.

Adulterants: *Umonia acidissima* Correa, *Garcinia mangostina* L. and *Puilica granatum* L. are used as substitute of *Aegle marmelos* Correa.

ALLIUM SATIVUM L. (ALLIACEAE)

English name: Garlic.

Sanskrit names: Arishta, Lashuna, Mahausada, Rason.

Vernacular names Asm : Naharu; **Ben:** Rasun; **Guj** : Lasan, Shunam; **Hin** : Lashun; **Kan** : Belluli; **Kon :** Lossun; **Mar:** Velluli, Velluthulli; **Mar:** Lasun; **Ori** : Rasun; **Tam:** Vellaipundu; **Tel:** Tellagadda.

Trade names: Rasun, Lashun.

Traditional use : *UPAVARHANA SAMHITA* : good for health; *AGNI PURANA:* a mixture of this plant, ginger and *Moringa oleifera* is helpful for eye and also as eardrop.

MATSYA PURANA : of great medicinal value, should be stored in forts.

UNANI: an ingredient of 'Seer (Lahsan) '.

HOMOEOPATHY: Mother tincture, a good remedy for cough and cold, pain in the chest, swelling of glands, *psoas, iliacus* and erosion of old diseases at the adimanic stage.

Modern use: *Bulb:* antidiabetic, antiinflammatory, anticancer, effective in rheumatism, catarrhal conditions; *Raw garlic:* decreases glucose, cholesterol, phospholipids, triglycerides, useful in dyspepsia, cryptococcal meningitis, rickettsia; applied externally as resolvent to indolent tumours, internally given with common salt in nervous diseases, headache;*Liniment:* beneficial in infantile convulsion and other spasmodic affections; *Juice:* applied to bruises and sprain, relieves earache, allays pain in otorrhoea; preparation have been given to pulmonary phthisis, bronchitis, gangrene of the lung and whooping cough; *Garlic juice:* good for treatment of laryngeal tuberculosis, lupus and duodenal ulcer; *Inhalation of fresh garlic juice:* useful in pulmonary tuberculosis, dyspep-sia, flatulence and colic; in external application, the *juice* is used as a rubifacient; in skin diseases, as an eyedrop and in earache.

Phytography : Hardy perennial bulbous scapigerous herb; stem flat, dry, lower portion of the plant forms bulb which consists of several smaller bulbs called *cloves,* surrounded by a thin white or pinkish sheath; leaves flat, narrow green; heads bear small white flowers and bulbils.

Phenology: *Flowering* and *Fruiting:* Winter.

Distribution: Cultivated throughout India since ancient days; also cultivated in Pakistan, Bangladesh and almost in all tropical countries.

Ecology and cultivation: It favours a richer soil and higher elevation (1000-1300 m), well-drained, moderately clayey loam is best suited for cultivation; requires a cool, moist period during growth and a relatively dry period during maturing of the crop; takes 4-5 months to mature, harvested during February to April. Yields good results, if treated with farmyard manure and top-dressing of ammonium sulphate mixed with superphosphate. It grows as a late irrigated crop; in South India, it is rotated with ragi.

Chemical contents: *Garlic:* protein 6. 3%, fat 0. 1 %, carbohydrate 29%, Ca 0. 03%, Fe 1. 3 mg/100 g, vitamin C 13 mg/100 g, and also Cu-peptides, 2 mercapto-L-cysteins, anthocyanins, glycosides of kaempferol and quercetin, polysaccharides, allinase, sterols, hydrocarbons, alliin (nonvolatile sulpher amino acid), sativin I & II, scordinines A & B; *Essential oil:* the bulbs, on distillation, yield 0. 06-0. 1 % of an essential oil containing allyl-propyl-disulphide, diallyl disulphide and two sulphur containing compounds.

ALOE BARBADENSIS MILL. (LILIACEAE)

Syn : *Aloe indica* Royle, *A. littoralis* Koening., *A. vera* Tourn. ex Linn.

English names: Barbados aloe, Curacas aloe, Indian aloe, Jafarabad aloe.

Sanskrit name: Ghritakumari.

Vernacular names: Asm : Chalkunwari; **Ben:** Ghritakumari; **Guj** : Kumarpathu, Kunvar; **Hin** : Ghee kunvar; **Kan** : Lolesara; **Kon** : Kantikkor, Katkunvor; **Mal:** Kattarvazha kumari; **Mar:** Korphad; **Ori** : Gheokunri; **Pun:** Ghikur, Kawargandal; **Tam:** Alagai, Chirukuttali, Kuttilai; **Tel:** Chinnakata banda, Kala banda, Kittanara.

Trade names: Ghritakumari, Ghee kunvar.

Traditional use: *TRIBAL: Leaf-pulp:* in liver troubles, jaundice, fever, gonorrhoea, spleen disorder, rheumatism, piles, dysmenorrhoea, sterility in women; *Leaf-mucilage:* mild laxative, to cure hardening of breast tissues, in insect stings.

AYURVEDA: alternative, bitter, cooling, purgative, sweet, tonic, anthelmintic, useful in eye diseases, tumours, enlargement of spleen, liver troubles, vomiting, skin diseases, bilious-ness, asthma, leprosy, jaundice, strangury, ulcer; *Flowers:* anthelmintic.

UNANI: Gheekawar is useful in inflammation of spleen, lumbago, muscular pain, ophthal-mia, digestive, purgative; *Leaves* good for piles and biliousness.

Modern use: *Aloe:* in menstrual diseases, stomach pain, tonic after pregnancy, uterine disorders, high fever; *Pulp:* menstrual suppressions, nervous imbalance; *Aloe com-pound:* in treatment of women sterility; *Mucilage:* painful inflammation; *Root:* colic pain; *Aloe mixture with other plant extracts:* for treating obstruction of lymphatic system.

Phytography : A coarse-looking plant with a short (30-60 cm high) stem; leaves succulent, green, large (37 cm long, 10 cm broad, 2 cm thick), densely crowded; flowers in racemes, bright yellow, tubular, stamens frequently projected beyond the perianth tube.

Phenology: *Flowering:* September-December; *Fruiting:* scarce.

Distribution: A native of North Africa, Canary Islands and Spain; naturalised in India; many varieties are found in a semi-wild state in all parts of India; also cultivated in pots and gardens.

Ecology and cultivation: Xerophyte; propagated by suckers.

Chemical contents: *Plant:* aloin, aloe-emodin and resins.

Adulterant: *Aloe candelabrum* Berger is used as substitute for *Aloe barbadensis* Miller.

ALSTONIA SCHOLARIS R. BR. (APOCYNACEAE)

Syn : *Echites scholaris* L., *E. pala* Ham.

English names: Devil's tree, Dita bark.

Sanskrit names: Saptaparni, Saptaparna, Sarada, Vishalalvaka, Vishamachhda, Ayugmaparna, Gandhiparna, Payasya, Jivani, Kshalrya, Madagandha, Grahashi, Grahanashana.

Vernacular names: Asm : Chatiar; **Ben:** Chhatim; **Hin** : Chatian, Salni chatian; **Kan** : Saptaparna, Maddale, Kodale, Elele kale, Janthalla, Hale; **Ken:** SantnarUkh; **Mal:** Ezhilampala, Mukkampala, Pala; **Mar:** Salvin; **Ori** : Chhatiana, Chhanchania; Silgandha; **Pun:** Satona; **Sin:** Rukattana; **Tam:** Elilaipillai, Mukumpalei, Pala, Wedrase; **Tel:** Eda kula, Pala garuda.

Trade names: Chatiyan, Shaitan wood, Saptaparni.

Traditional use: *MUNDAS OF CHOTANAGPUR* : *Bark:* in colic pain; *SOME PARTS OF INDIA: Plant:* used in the treatment of leprosy; *Twig:* hung in the room of the newly confined woman to lessen the activities of evil spirit on the new born.

ATHARVA VEDA: preventive and curative of diseases caused by change of season. *CHARAKA SAMHITA* and *SUSHRUTA SAMHITA:* good for headache, sores, and some other diseases; *A YURVEDA* : the following uses are recommended: (i) *Bark:* dermal sores, ragging fever, discharge of sperm with urine, hiccup, insufficiency in breast milk, gout, cold congestion, dyspepsia; (ii) *Latex:* caries, pimple, pyorrhoea; (iii) *Flower:* asthma, respiratory troubles.

UNANI: Ingredient of 'Kashim'.

HOMOEOPATHY: Malarial fever, anaemia, indigestion, general debility and other stomach ailments.

Modern use: *Bark:* known in commerce as *Dita bark* and is used in medicine as bitter, febrifuge and astringent, in treatment of malarial fever, chronic dysentery, diarrhoea and in snake bite; *Milky juice:* applied to ulcers.

Phytography: Large (20 m high, 3 m girth), evergreen tree with straight, often fluted and buttressed base, branches whorled, bark yellow inside and exudes milky bitter latex; leaves simple, whorled-usually 7 in a whorl, coriaceous, whitish beneath, obovate or elliptic or oblong, obtuse rounded or obtusely acuminate, 30-60 pairs of horizontal veins joining an intramarginal one; cymes peduncled or sessile, umbellately branched; flowers aromatic, 0. 8-1. 25 cm in diameter, greenish white, pubescent; follicles 30-60 cm long and 0. 3 cm in diameter, pendulous, in clusters.

Phenology: *Flowering:* Autumn; *Fruiting:* Winter.

Distribution: Throughout moist regions of India, especially in West Coast forests, in the Himalaya it ascends up to 1000 m; also found in Bangladesh and Pakistan. Planted in the gardens.

Ecology and cultivation: Also grown as an ornamental.

Adulterants: *Alstonia macrophylla* Wall. and A. *venenata* R. Br. are used as substitute for A. *scholaris.*

ANACARDIUM OCCIDENTALE L. (ANACARDIACEAE)

English name: Cashew nut.

Vernacular names: Asm : Kaju badam; **Ben**: Hijli badam, Kaju badam; **Guj**, **Hin**, **Mar** and **Pun**: Kaju; **Kan** : Gerupappu; Godambi; **Kon**: Kaz; **Mat**: Kashumaru, Parankimara, Andiparuppau; **Ori** : Lanka badam; **Tam**: Mundiri, Munthirikai; **Tel**: Jidimamidi, Muntha mamidi.

Trade names: Cashew nut, Kaju.

Traditional use: *Cashew nut shell-oil:* mild purgative, used in folk medicine for treatment of hookworm, cracks on soles of feet, warts, corns, leporus sores.

Modern use: *Cashew nut:* used in mental derangement, sexual debility, nervous prostration following seminal emission, morning sickness in pregnancy, palpitation of heart, rheumatic percarditis, loss of memory as a sequel to small pox; *Kernel:* good for week

patients suffering from I incessant and chronic vomiting;*Kernel-oil:* antidote for irritant poisons; *Liquor made from fruit:* diuretic.

HOMOEOPATHY : for boils, warts, wounds and different types of cracks in legs; used sometimes in case of leprosy.

Phytography : Small tree with short, thick, crooked trunk; leaves simple, alternate, petiolate, entire, hard, 10-20 cm by 7. 5-12. 5 cm; panicles terminal, bracteate, pubescent; branches long, naked to the tips, flowers yellow with pink stripes, 0. 8 cm in diameter; cashew apple red or yellow-is the swollen, enlarged pedicel which bears the nut.

Phenology: *Flowering:* March-April; *Fruiting:* April-May.

Distribution: Native to tropical America, naturalised in the hotter sea-shores of India; Pakistan, Bangladesh and Malaysia.

Ecology and cultivation: Introduced; grows in plains, especially towards the coast, very occasionally ascending up to 1200 m; being extensively planted by clearing scrub jungles in the plains.

Chemical contents: *Bark:* exudes gum; *Flower:* polyphenols; *Cashew shell:* yields gum, oil and liquid (CNSL); *Liquid-free nutshell:* syringic and gallic acids, galocatechin; *Defatted nutshell:* naringenin, prunin-6"-O-p-coumarate;

Cashew apple liquor: vitamin C, vitamin E; *Reddish brown testa:* D-catechin, gallic acid, caffeic acid, quinic acid, polyphenols, bioflavone.

ANDROGRAPHIS PANICULATA (BURM. F.) WALL. EX NEES (ACANTHACEAE)

Syn : *Justicia paniculata* Burm. f.

English names: The great king of bitters, the creat. Sanskrit names: Bhunimba, Kirata.

Vernacular names: Ben: Kalmegh; **Guj :** Kariyatu; **Hin:** Kirayat; **Kan:** Nelabaru; **Mar:** Olikiryata; **Tam** and **Tel:** Nelavemu.

Trade names: Kalmegh, Kirayat.

Traditional use: *Plant:.* febrifuge, alterative, anthelmintic, anodyne, useful in debility, diabetes, consumption, influenza, bronchitis, itches and piles; in Bengal, household medicine known as 'Kalmegh', made from leaves, is given to the children suffering from stomach complaints.

HOEMOEPATHY: used for treatment of different ailments of head, mind, eyes, nose, mouth, tongue, throat, abdomen, stool, urine, fever and other modalities.

Modern use: *Drug constitute stem, leaf* and *inflorescence:* as a tonic and in the treatment of fevers, worms, dysentery and also beneficial to liver and digestive ailments; it is reported that it has some antityphoid and antibiotic activity; *Decoction:* used for sluggishness of liver and in jaundice.

Phytography : An erect herb with square stem, glabrous below, glandular hairy above; leaves linear, lanceolate, glabrous and distinctly pedicelled; flowers white or pale purple; capsules compressed transversely; seeds bony.

Phenology: *Flowering* and *Fruiting:* September-May.

Distribution: Throughout India in the plains and hills; Bangladesh, Pakistan, all South- East Asian and SAARC countries.

Ecology and cultivation: Common in stony lines in forests and in wastelands. Culti-vated as an ornamental.

Chemical contents: *Plant:* kalmeghin, bitter principle andrographolide; bitterness is due to nonbasic principle.

Adulterants: It is used as adulterants for *Chirata,* and is a substitute for quinine.

Remark: Whole plant is bitter.

ABROMA AUGUSTA (L) LT. (STERCULIACEAE)

(now known as *Ambroma* L. f.)

Syn : *Abroma augulata* Lam., A. *wheeleri* Retz., A. *fastuosum* Gaertn., *Theobroma augusta* L.

English name: Devil's cotton.

Vernacular names: Asm : Bon kopashi; **Hin** and **Ben:** Ulat kambal; **Tam:** Sivapputtutti.

Trade name: Ulat kambal.

Traditional use: *Seed:* yields fatty oil, rich in linoleic acid and lowers cholesterol level in blood.

HOMOEOPATHY : used to control mind, different ailments of head, heart, eyes, ears, nose, face, mouth, throat, stomach, abdomen, urinary organs, male and female sexual organs, respiratory organs, neck, back and limbs, skin diseases, fever; to regulate appetite and sleep.

Modern use: *Fresh* and *dried root-bark:* used as uterine tonic and emmenagogue; regulates menstrual flow; *Fresh juice from root-bark:* useful in congestive and neuralgic forms of dysmenorrhoea, amenorrhoea, urinary trouble, bronchitis, broncho-pneumonia, carbuncles and poisonous boils; *Leaf:* used in diabetes, rheumatic pain and sinusitis.

Phytography : Shrub, branches downy; leaf simple, cordate, 10-15 cm by 10-12. 5 cm, base 3-7 costate, repand-denticulate while the upper narrower leaves are entire, glabrescent above and tomentose below, petiolate, petioles 1. 25-2. 5 cm long, stipules linear, as long as the petiole, deciduous; flowers axillary, pedunculate, peduncle 3. 5 cm long; capsules 5-angled, 5-winged, obpyramidal, thrice as long as the persistent calyx; seeds albuminous, numerous.

Distribution: Widely distributed in hotter parts of India up to 1500 m; Bangladesh, Pakistan and the adjacent countries.

Ecology and cultivation: Plant prefers hot and moist climate; sometimes planted, occasionally found as an escape.

Chemical contents: *Plant:* fixed oil, a little resinous matter, alkaloid (minute quantity) and water-soluble bases.

ACANTHUS ILICIFOLIUS L. (ACANTHACEAE)

Syn : *Acanthus doloarius* Blanco, *Dilivaria ilicifolia* Nees

Sanskrit name: Harikasa.

Vernacular names: Ben: Hargoza, Harkachkanta; **Kan** : Holeculli; **Mal**: Payinaculli; **Mar**: Maranda, Maraneli; **Ori** : Harkamcli; **Tam**: Kalutai mulli; **Tel**: Alei.

Trade name: Harkasa.

Traditional use: *TRIBES OF SUNDARBANS: Root* (boiled in mustard oil) : in paralysis of limbs; *FOLKS OF GOA: Leaf:* as fomentation in rheumatism and neuralgia.

Modern use: *Plant:* in asthma; *Decoction of plant:* in dyspepsia; *Leaf* and *tender shoot:* in snake bite; *Root:* in asthma, paralysis, leucorrhoea and debility; *Leaf:* as fomentation in rheumatism, neuralgia and in snake bite.

Phytography : Erect herb; stems up to 1. 5 m, in clumps, little divided, glabrous; leaves shortly petioled, oblong or elliptic, base usually spinous, toothed or, pinnatifid, rigid, glabrous; spikes 10-40 cm, terminal, commonly solitary; flowers mostly opposite, bract and bracteoles present, sepals 4, outer 2 elliptic rounded, inner 2 broadly lanceolate, subacute, petals 5, blue, united, 2-lipped, corolla tube short, pubescent within, stamens 4, didynamous, shorter than coroll_ lip, filaments stout, anthers 1-lobed, bearded, carpels 2, united, ovary 2-chambered having 2 ovules in chamber, style short, bifid; capsules shining chestnut-brown, ellipsoid, compressed, 0. 6-0. 8 cm long; testa white, very lax.

Phenology: *Flowering* and *Fruiting:* almost throughout the year.

Distribution: Mangroves of Indian peninsula; Sri Lanka, Bangladesh, Pakistan and the adjoining areas.

Ecology and cultivation: Commonly grown on the river banks, tidal canal sides, low swampy areas in the mangrove forests and its vicinity; wild.

Chemical contents: *Plant:* acanthicifoline, oleanolic acid, â-sitosterol, lupeol, quercetin and its glucopyranoside, trigonellin; *Root:* saponin, glycoside of 3á-OH-lup-20(29) -ene.

ACONITUM FEROX WALL. (RANUNCULACEAE)

Syn: *Aconitum virosum* Don., A. *napellus* var. *rigidum* Hook, f & T.

English names: Wolf's bane, Indian aconite.

Sanskrit names: Vatsanabha, Visa.

Vernacular names: Hin: Bish, Mahoor; **Guj** and **Mar:** Vachang; **Kas:** Mohra; **Tam:** Vasnumbi; **Tel:** Vasnabhi.

Trade name: Bish.

Traditional use: *AYURVEDA* : *Root:* used in the *mrityunjaya rasa* (used to treat the fever supposed to be caused by deranged *vayu,* i.e., wind, *sannipatika jvara,* i.e., remittent fever, *hinguleswarc-rasa, anandabhairav agnitundi vati,* etc.

Vatsanabha has been used in medicine from a very remote period. It is regarded as healing and stimulant. It is used in a great variety of affections, but is specially recommended in fever, cephalagia, affections of throat, dyspepsia and rheumatism. *HOMOEOPATHY:* remedy for clotting of blood in heart or in lungs, pneumonia, Iymptisis, pleurisy, eye trouble, earache, toothache and urinary trouble.

Modern use: Extremely poisonous; used in leprosy, fever, cholera, nasal catarrah, tonsillitis, sore throat, gastric disorders, debility, etc., also used as a sedative and diaphoretic; applied in the form of paste in cases of neuralgia and rheumatism.

Phytography : Perennial erect herb growing up to 2 m in height; roots look like the navel of children; leaves alternate, simple, rounded or oval, may be palmately 5-lobed; flowers borne on branched racemes, bracts and bracteoles present, large helmet-type, helmet vaulted with short sharp beak, pale dirty blue in colour, zygomorphic, floral parts arranged spirally on an elongated receptacle; follicles erect, usually densely villose-sometimes glabrous.

Phenology: *Flowering* and *Fruiting:* July-November.

Distribution : Alpine Himalaya including Nepal; *endemic.*

Ecology and cultivation: Temperate to alpine regions of the Himalaya in the altitude of 3300-5000 m.

Chemical contents: *Root:* pseudoaconitine (a toxic alkaloid), indactonitine, chasmaconitine, bikhaconitine.

Adulterants: Indian aconite root is known as 'bikh' or 'bish', the name which is applied to aconite from more than one species, and different authors have ascribed it to different species.

Remarks: *Vulnerable* due to excessive collection for medicinal uses. Collection in wild state should be banned and measures for cultivation should be initiated.

ACORUS CALAMUS L. (ARACEAE)

Syn : *Acorus griffithii* Schott., A. *belangeii* Schott, A. *casia* Bertol.

English name: The sweet flag.

Sanskrit name: Vacha.

Vernacular names: Asm, **Ben** and **Hin** : Boch; **Gui** : Godavaj, Vekhand; **Kan** : Baje, Baje gida; **Kon:** Waikhand; **Mal:** Vayambu; **Mar:** Vekhand; **Ori** : Bacha; **Pun:** Bari, Boj, Warch; **Tam:** Vasamboo; **Tel:** Vasa.

Trade name: Boch.

Traditional Use

Santal **:** Use the plant in the following ways: (i) they mix and grind black pepper, cloves, root of *Carissa carandus* lo along with little of the rootstock of A. *calamus* lo, then stir the same in pure mustard oil-the emulsion, thus prepared is anointed daily over the whole body of the patient suffering form epilepsy with foaming and groaning, as soon as the fit comes on; a few drops of this emulsion should be poured into the nose of the patient; (ii) for the treatment of indigestion, they take pills made by grinding 100 black peppers, little amount of ginger and the root of A. *calamus* together; (iii) also use in the treatment of asthma, bronchitis, cold and cough, dry cough, epilepsy, haemopty-sis, indigestion, phthisis; *BIRHOR* : *Rhizome* in alopecia, *Root* as massage, in fever, hysteria, pain in neck, teething trouble of children, malaria and cancer.

Agni Purana : This plant is of great medicinal value; it recommends the following uses: (i) for treatment of epilepsy, this plant should be boiled with *Costus speciosus, shankhapushpi,* along with the juice of *Bacopa monnieri;* the substance thus obtained should be administered to the patient; (ii) drinking the decoction of this plant, *Piper peepuloides, Staphyles emodi* Wall., and *Cyperus parviflorus* Heyne and *pippalimula* is good for the patient of rheumatic arthritis; (iii) the powder or decoction of this plant helps curing chronic enlargement of spleen; (iv) decoction of the plant is beneficial for the patient of dropsy; *A YURVEDA: Rhizome:* bitter, healing, emetic, laxative, diuretic, carminative; improves voice and appetite; good for oral diseases, abdominal pain, epilepsy, bronchitis, hysteria, loss of memory, rat bite and worms in ear.

***Siddha System*:** Fresh root for bronchial asthma.

Unani: An ingredient of the medicine called 'Waje-Turki'; useful in flatulent colic, chronic dyspepsia, catarrhal, in burn wounds, carminative, anthelmintic and as bitter tonic.

Modern use: *Rhizome:* aromatic, bitter, carminative, emetic, stimulant, stomachic, useful in dyspepsia, colic, remittent fevers, nerve tonic, in bronchitis, dysentery, epilepsy and other mental ailments, glandular and abdominal tumours and in snake bite.

Phytography: Perennial, erect, aromatic herb, common on river banks and marshes, ascending to 3000 m; rhizome cylindrical or slightly compressed, about 2. 5 cm in diameter, much-branched, externally light brown or pinkish brown but white and spongy within; leaves distichous, large, 1-2 m in length, base equitant, margin waved; spadix sessile, cylindric, densely flowered, not completely enclosed by spathe, spathe 15-75 cm in length, narrow, leaf-like; flowers small, bisexual; berries few-seeded; seeds oblong, albuminous.

Phenology: *Flowering* and *Fruiting:* July-August; fruiting very rare.

Distribution: Throughout India; ascending the Himalaya up to 2000 m; Sri Lanka, Pakistan and Bangladesh.

Ecology and cultivation: Probably introduced; found from the coast to 1200 m; often near village wells and along watercourses; confined to marshy areas; gregarious herb from a stout horizontal rhizome; wild and cultivated.

Chemical contents: *Dry rhizome* :1. 5-3. 5% of a yellow aromatic volatile oil-calamus oil; the oil contains â-asarone, small quantities of sesquiterpenes and sesquiterpenes alcohols; *Rhizome:* also contains choline (0. 26%), flavone, acoradin, 2, 4, 5-tri-MeO-benzaldehyde, 2, 5-di-MeO-benzoquinone, galangin, calameone, acolamone, isoacolamone, epoxyisoacoragermacrone; *Aerial parts:*

lutcolin-6, 8-c-diglucoside; chemical constituents vary in ecotypes and polyploides.

Adulterants: The powdered drug has been adulterated with siliceous earth, ground marsh mallow root and cereal flowers.

Remark: Rhizomes are valued for indigenous medicine.

ARECA CATECHU L. (ARECACEAE)

English names: Areca palm, Areca nut, Betel nut, Pinang palm.

Sanskrit names: Gubak, Phalam, Poag, Pooga, Poogi.

Vernacular names: Asm : Tambul; **Ben**: Supari, Gua; **Guj** : Supaari; **Hin** : Kasaili,

Supari; **Kan** : Adike, Bette; **Kon** : Maddi; **Mal**: Adakka, Pugam, Pakka; **Mar**: Supari **Ori** : Gua; **Tam**: Kamubu, Pakku; **Tel**: Poke, Vakka.

Trade names: Areca nut, Betel nut, Supari. There are over 150 trade types.

Traditional use: *SANTAL:* (i) a patient of small pox is given to eat the areca nut when the pustules subside; (ii) a mixture for biliary colic is prepared with areca nut as a constituent; (iii) an ointment for chancre and syphilis is made by pestling areca nut with the root of *Gymnema hirsutus,* leaf of *Piper betel* and then cooking the same in mustard oil or butter; *TRIBALS* also use this plant in rhagadas, venereal sores, syphilis, dysentery, cholera, small pox and for fractured bones.

References to this plant are found in the *BHAGVA* TA along with the plants of Musa paradisica and *Borassus flabellifer. CHARAKA SAMHITA* : *Fruit:* useful in the diseases caused by bile; *SUSHRUTA SAMHITA* : *Fruit:* beneficial in the diseases caused by phlegm; but overuse of this may distort voice of a man; *CHACRADATTA* : *Paste of unripe fruit:* may be used as liniment; *Extract of unripe fruit:* useful in small pox; *HARITA SAMHITA* : sesame oil in which extract of unripe fruit has been boiled should be used; *A YURVEDA* : various preparations of *unripe* and *ripe nuts* are useful in toothache, pyorrhea, gum diseases, in treatment of worms, while *extract of young leaf* mixed with mustard oil is useful as liniment in rheumatism; *BRAHMAVAIVARTA PURANA* : brushing the teeth with twig of this plant is beneficial; *AGNI PURANA* : (i) immortality can be attained by consuming decoction of this plant along with the powder of root, bark, leaf and fruit of margosa and juice of *Wedelia calendulacea;* (ii) alkaloids of this plant are beneficial medicine.

UNANI: Ingradient of 'Futal (Chalia)'.

Modern use: *Nut:* chewing facilitates salivation, it being a good source of fluoride prevents tooth decay, but constant use might cause oral carcinoma; shows antimicrobial activities; *Aqueous extract of nut:* exhibits vascoconstriction and adrenalin p. Qtentiation in rats; *Extract of leaf* and *fruit:* spasmogenic.

Phytography : Tall, slender, unbranched palm with a crown of leaves; stem annulate; leaves pinnate with a conspicuous sheet; flowers in spadix, male many at the upper portion, female much longer and a few at the base; fruits are single-seeded berries with flesh and fibrous pericarp and a stony seed, 3. 8-5 em long, smooth, orange or scarlet when ripe.

Phenology: *Flowering:* August-January; *Fruiting:* about a year later.

Distribution: Cultivated in the coastal regions of India, Bangladesh, Pakistan, Sri Lanka, Myanmar and other tropical and subtropical countries.

Ecology and cultivation: This palm requires a moist tropical climate with heavy (500 cm/year) rainfall provided with good drainage. It can be grown in drier areas (rainfall 50 cm/year), if properly irrigated. It is a shade-loving plant, especially in the earlier stages and is very sensitive to drought. It grows on a variety of soils, but saline or alkaline soil, light and sandy soil are not suitable for it, but slightly saline sandy soil is good.

It is generally cultivated as a mixed crop with coconut and plantain or along with *Erythrina indica.* The betel nuts are sown in October/November with a distance of 10-15 em between two nuts. Transplanting is normally done after two years, occasionally after 3 or 4 years. Transplantation is done in July in the highlands and from February to April in lowlands. The second transplantation takes place when the first have come into bearing. In a fully planted grove, a distance of about 2 m each way is kept between the betel nut tree.

Chemical contents: *Nut:* alkaloids-arecoline, arecaidine, guvacine and isoguvacine.

Adulterants: Fruits of *Areca triandra* Roxb. and *Areca nagensis* Griff. are substitutes for *Areca catechu* L.

Remark: Stem and leaves are used in various ways. vascoconstriction and adrenalin p. Qtentiation in rats; *Extract of leaf* and *fruit:* spasmogenic.

ARISTOLOCHIA INDICA L. (ARISTOLOCHIACEAE)

English name: Indian birthwort.

Sanskrit name: Ishvari.

Verṇacular names: Ben and **Hin** : Isharmul; **Mal:** Isvaramuli; **Mar:** Sapasan; **Tel:** Eswaramuli.

Trade name: Iswarmul.

Traditional use: *Root:* tonic, stimulant, emetic, emmenagogue, in fever, in powder form is given with honey for leucoderma; *Root-decoction:* in impotency; *Crushed root:* applied on itching; *Juice of leaf:* in snake bite, used for cough; *Seed:* inflammations, biliousness and dry cough.

UNANI: a constituent of 'Majnoon-e-Flasfa'.

Modern use: *Plant:* used as abortifacient; *EtOH* (50%) *extract:* diuretic and anti-inflammatory; *Dried stem* and *root:* used as drug, which should be used in minimal doses; the drug promotes digestion and controls menstruation; in higher doses, it may prove lethal, it is used as a stimulant, tonic and for fevers; in moderate doses, it is used as a gastric stimulant and in dyspepsia; *Root:* considered as a stimulant, tonic and emmenagogue and also used in intermittent fever and in bowl troubles of children; shows antifertility activity in experimental animals.

Phytography : Twining herb, semiwoody, having more or less swollen nodes; leaves cordate or ovate, exstipulate; flowers irregular, often offensively smelling, perianth globose with a purple dilated and trumpet-shaped mouth with a strap-shaped brown purple appendage or lip behind; fruit a subglobose capsule.

Phenology: *Flowering:* June to October; *Fruiting:* November to March.

Distribution: Found throughout the subcontinent, mainly in the plains and lower hilly regions from Nepal to Bangladesh.

Ecology and cultivation: Found in open scrub jungles; wild.

Chemical contents: *Root:* a crystalline substance-probably a glucoside, a micro-crys-talline principle glucosidic in nature named isoaristolochic acid, allantoin, 0. 05% carbonyl compounds and a small amount of an oil, with the odour of isovanillin, ishwarone, ishwarane, aristolochene.

ASPARAGUS RACEMOSUS WILLD. VAR. *JAVANICUS* BAKER (LILIACEAE)

Syn : *Asperagus tetragonus.*

English name: Asparagus.

Sanskrit names: Shatavari, Shatamuli.

Vernacular names: Asm : Shatamul; **Ben:** Shatamuli; **Guj** : Satawari; **Hin** : Shakakul, Sada bori, Shatamuli, Satwar; **Mal:** Shatavali; **Mar:** Shatavari, Shatavarimul; **Ori** : Shatamuli; **Tam:** Chattavari, Cadumullam, Shimai shadavari; **Tel** :Challagadda.

Trade names: Shatamuli, Asparagus.

Traditional use: *SOME TRIBES OF INDIA: Root:* refrigerant, antiseptic, alterative and galactogogue; roots form a constituent of medicinal oils used for nervous and rheumatic complaints; powder boiled with milk and sugar has been used in different types of neurological disorders, urinary calculi; rub the root of the plant in different diseases of urinary organs; *Powder of leaf:* enhances breast milk, used for the treatment of colon syndrome.

AYURVEDA : useful in different types of cardiac abnormality; beneficial for intelligence as well as on memory modulatory; *Powder of root* (boiled with milk) : for treatment of night blindness; .

UNANI : Ingredient of 'Satawar'.

Modern use: *Root:* used as demulcent, aphrodisiac, diuretic, antidysenteric, in impotency, azoospermea.

Phytography : A slender, scrambling/scandent suffruticose perennial, woody, prickly shoots with reflexed spines; cladode more or less acicular and triquetrous falcate 13-26 mm long; divaricate, finely acuminate; flowers white, sweet-scented, :t 6 mm on filiform articulate pedicels, 6-12 mm long in very short racemes; berries 2. 5-6 mm in diameter, scarlet, red on ripening.

Phenology: *Flowering:* September-December; deciduous or dying back to the root in the hot season; *Fruiting:* throughout the year.

Distribution: Throughout tropical and subtropical regions of the country,

Ecology and cultivation: Common in scrub jungles and in forests; cultivated as ornamentals.

Chemical contents: *Leaf:* quercetin-3-glucoronide, sitosterol, stigmasterol, sarsasapogenin, sito-sterol D-glucoside, stigmasterol-B-D-glucoside, two sirostanolic and two furostandic saponins.

Remark: Root is used in veterinary medicine.

BACOPA MONNIERI (L.) PENNEL (SCROPHULARIACEAE)

Syn: *Herpestis monniera* (L.) H. B. & K., *Moniera cuneifolia* Michx., *Gratiola monniera* L.

English name: Thyme leaved gratiola.

Sanskrit names: Brahmi, Nira brahmi.

Vernacular names: Ben: Adhabirni, Birmi shak, Barmi shak, Brahmi; **Hin** : Barambhi, Safed chammi; **Mal:** Nir bramhi; **Mar:** Barna; **Ori** : Urishnaparni; Tam: Nirbrami; **Tel:** Sambranichettu.

Trade name: Brahmi.

Traditional use: *ATHARVA VEDA:* strengthens body, improves quality of semen; *CHARAKA SAMHITA* : invigorat-ing, life sustaining; *SUSHRUTA SAMHITA* : increases memory and lifespan; *AYURVEDA:* (a) *Plant:* bitter, diuretic, blood-purifier, invigorates sex; (b) *Plant-extract:* used in purification of blood, for anaemia, dermatitis, diabetes, filaria; (c) *Plant-juice* (along with ginger, sugar and bark extract of *Moringa oleifera*) : to children in stomach disorder; (d) *Leaves* (fried in *ghee)* : as a brain tonic, in nervous weakness, hysteria, epilepsy, insanity, anxiety neurosis, and to sharpen dull memory.

AGNI PURANA: Plant: poison-killer; *Plant-juice:* good for epilepsy. *UNANI:* invigorating and good for cold and cough.

Modern use: *Plant-extract:* In experiments with mice, rat and dog, it has been proved to be tranquilizer, musculature relaxant, antispasmodic, anticancer; *Powdered dried leaf:* satisfactory results obtained in man in cases of asthenia, nervous breakdown, and other low adynamic conditions.

Phytography : Annual creeper, rooting at each node; stem soft, succulent, soft hairs present; branches 10-25 cm long; leaves alternate, simple, 1. 25-1. 8 cm long, sessile or subsessile, oval-shaped; flowers light blue or white, 0. 8-1. 5 cm long; capsules 2-grooved, valves separating from entire column, many-seeded.

Phenology: *Flowering:* April-June; *Fruiting:* June-December.

Distribution: Marshes throughout India, ascending up to 1300 m; Bangladesh, Pakistan and Sri Lanka.

Ecology and cultivation: Grows in damp or marshy areas, on the banks of ponds and canals, in the crop fields.

Chemical contents: *Plant:* Becoside A & B, betulic acid, betulinic acid, d-mannitol, stigmasterol, â-sitosterol, saponin, stigmastanol, hersaponin, monnierin, nicotine, luteoline and its glucosides.

BALANITES AEGYPTICA (L.) DELILE (BALANITACEAE)

Syn : *Balanites roxburghii* Planch, *B. aegyptica* var. *roxburghii* Duthie.

English names: Desert date, Soapberry tree, Thorn tree.

Sanskrit name: Ingudi.

Vernacular names: Ben and **Hin** : Hingan; **Mar:** Hinganbet; **Tam:** Nanjunda; **Tel:** Gari.

Trade name: Hingan.

Traditional use : *TRIBES OF PANCH MAHAL* (Maharashtra) and *RURAL FOLK: Bark, Leaf, Fruit* and *Seed:* as anthelmintic and purgative; *Fruit:* in boils, leucoderma and other skin diseases; *Fruit-pulp:* in whooping cough.

Modern use: *Plant:* cytotoxic and antitumour principle isolated; *Bark:* bactericide; *EtOH (50%) extract of bark:* spasmolytic; *Seed-kernel oil:* antimicrobial, useful in burns and ulcers, spermicidal.

Phytography : Spiny tree, about 6 m high; branches glabrous or puberulous and ending in very strong ascending spines; leaves alternate, bifoliate, ashy green, leaflets coriaceous; cymes axillary, 4-to 10-flowered; flowers green, velvety pubescent; fruits ovoid, about 5 cm in length, fleshy drupes, 1-seeded; seed oily but exalbuminou8

Phenology: *Flowering:* November, also during February to May; *Fruiting:* Winter.

Distribution: Bihar, Deccan, Gujarat, Uttar Pradesh (Kanpur) and Sikkim.

Ecology and cultivation: Xerophyte, found chiefly on black cotton soil; does not thrive in rocky areas.

Chemical contents: *Plant:* diosgenin and yamogenin; *Root:* steroidal sapogenin, diosgenin, yamogenin; *Stem-bark:* steroidal sapogenin, nitrogen glucoside, sesquiterpene, balanitol, bergapten; *Leaf:* 6 diosgenin glucosides; *Fruit:* steroidal sapogenin, yamogenin, 5 diosgenin glycerides, 6 diosgenin glucosides, diosgenin, balanitisins A, B, C, D & E; *Seed:* a saponin of diosgenin, non-edible fatty oil.

Remarks: Fruit-pulp is edible and used for cleansing silk and cotton. Fruit-shell is used in fire-cracker industry. Wood is chiefly used for making walking sticks and as fuel.

BUTEA MONOSPERMA (LAMK.) TAUB. (FABACEAE)

Syn : *Butea frondosa* Roxb., *Erythrina monosperma* Lamk.

English names: Flame of the forest, Parrot tree.

Sanskrit name Palasha.

Vernacular names: Asm and **Ben:** Palash; **Guj** : Khakar; **Hin** : Dhak; **Kan** : Muttugathoras, Muttugu-mara; **Mal:** Chamath, Khakar; **Mar:** Palash; **Mun** : Murud ba; **Orn** : Murka; **Ori:** Palasa; . **Pun:** Dhak; **Sad:** Pal as, Paras; **Tam:** Samithu, Pal-asam; **Tel:** Moduga, Palashamu.

Trade names Palasha, Dhak.

Traditional use: *KHASI* and *GARO* : *Leaf:* in delirium; *TRIBES OF PURULIA* (West Bengal) : *Seed:* in ascaris; *TRIBES OF* MA *YURBHANJA* (Orissa) : *Seed:* as contraceptive; *TRIBES OF SANTAL PARGANAS* (Bihar) : *Root:* in tuberculosis; *TRIBES OF VARANASI* (Uttar Pradesh) : *Leaf:* in boils; *Seed:* as vermifuge; *TRIBES OF MIRZAPUR* (Uttar Pradesh) : *Bark:* in dysentery; *Gum:* in diarrhoea, dysentery; *TRIBES OF SIWALIK* (Uttar Pradesh) : *Gum:* as tonic; *BHAT: Seed:* as abortifacient; *BHOXA: Bark:* in bone fracture, *Gum:* in piles, urinary complaints; *GARHWALI: Leaf:* in boil, inflammation, *Flower:* in diarrhoea, dysentery, pimples, *Seed:* as anthelmintic; *THARU: Gum:* as diuretic, *Seed:* as cooling agent; *FOLKS OF DELHI: Gum:* as astringent, *Flower:* as aphrodisiac, astringent, diuretic, *Seed:* as anthelmintic; *FOLKS OF KURUKSHETRA* (Haryana) : *Flower:* in stomachache; *DANG: Bark:* in diarrhoea; *TRIBESOFRATANMAHAL HILLS* (Gujarat) : *Flower:* in eye complaints; *KORKU* (of Maharashtra) : *Flower,* in dysentery; *TRIBES OF KHANDLA* (Maharashtra) : *Flower:* in dog bite, urinary complaints; *TRIBES OF CHANDRAPURA* (Maharashtra) : *Leaf:* in skin diseases; *TRIBES OF JHABUA* (Madhya Pradesh) : *Root:* in dog bite; *TRIBES OF SAGAR* (Madhya Pradesh) : *Leaf:* as vermifuge, *Flower:* in diabetes, diarrhoea, piles; *TRIBES OF EAST GODAVARI* (Andhra Pradesh) : *Gum:* in diarrhoea; *TRIBES OF NILGIRI* (Tamil Nadu) : *Bark:* as haemostatic, in wounds, *Flower:* in eye complaints; *TRIBES OF KANNANORE* (Kerala) : *Flower:* in antifertility.

ATHARVA VEDA: Extract of stem: beneficial for sperms and helps securing conception; *CHARAKA SAMHITA : Stem-extract:* useful in leprosy, piles, gastroenteritis and menorrha-gia; *SUSHRUTA SAMHITA* : useful in diseases caused by *vayu* (wind), *Seed:* effective against intestinal worms; A *YURVEDA* : *Bark:* useful against snake venom, wounds, indigestion, gastroenteritis, fever, tuberculosis, *Gum:* astringent, beneficial to children and women, *Leaf:* astringent, sex stimulant, useful in intestinal worms, dyspepsia, piles, menorrhagia, pimples, wounds in mouth/throat, *Flower:* diuretic, sex stimulant, helps menstruation, useful in gastroenteritis, *Seed:* useful against intestinal worms.

SIDDHA : *Flower-juice:* used in preparation of the medicine *Murukkam, Seed* and *Kernel:* in *Palac*

UNANI: Ingredient of the medicine called 'Dhak(tesu) ' and 'Samaghke Dhak'.

Modern use: *Plant* (alcoholic extract: produces persistent vasodepression in cats, shows activity against earthworms; *Bark:* insecticide against house flies; *Alcohol extract of bark* : inhibitory against *E. coli* and *Micrococcus pyogenes* var. *aureus; Gum:* solution applied to check conception; *Root* (bark) : aphrodisiac, analgesic, anthelmintic, useful in elephan-tiasis, applied in sprue, piles, ulcers, tumours and dropsy; *EtOH* (50%) *extract of leaf:* spasmogenic; *FlolYer:* effective in leprosy, gout; *Alcoholic extract:* antiestrogenic in mice; *Aqueous extract:* anti-implantation in rats; along with *Hygrophila auriculata* leaf and root taken with milk to cure leucorrhoea; *Seed* (freshly powdered) : effective against Ascaris; *Extract (in vitro)* : anthelmintic against *Asacridia galli* worms; *finely powdered* along with *Acorus calamus* rhizome or mixed with juice of *Cyperus rotundus* rhizome: cures delirium; *Saline extract:* agglutinates erythrocytes of animals; *Hot alcoholic extract:* anti-implantation and anti-ovulatory in animals.

Phytography : Erect tree, reaching a height of 13-17 m; young stem clothed with grey or brown silky hairs; leaves alternate, petioles 7. 5-15. 0 cm long, trifoliate, leaflets 10-20 cm long, leathery, lower surface covered with dense silky hairs; racemes 15 cm long; flowers bright orange-red, thickly clothed on the outside with silvery small hairs; pods 15-20 cm by 3. 7-5. 0 cm, narrowed suddenly into a stalk longer than calyx.

Phenology: *Flowering:* February-April; *Fruiting:* May-July.

Distribution: Plains of India, ascending up to 1300 m; Myanmar.

Ecology and cultivation: Mesophyte; wild.

Chemical contents: *Plant:* flavonoids, glucosides, butin, butrin, isobutrin, palastrin; *Flower:* butrin, coriopsin, monospermoside, sulphurein, chalcones; *Seed:* palasonin, *Seed oil:* d-lactone of n-heneicosanoic acid, monospermine, new phytolectin.

Remarks: An important tree for lac cultivation, but the lac produced on it is of inferior quality. Bark yields fibre, wood yields timber of poor quality; stem-bark used as fish poison by tribes of South Rajasthan. Plates and bowls are made by stitching the leaves by the tribes of Purulia and Saurashtra. Flowers yield a yellow dye of little permanency.

Flowers are eaten as vegetables by tribes of Manbhum and Hazaribagh Districts of Bihar while fruits by Garhwalis.

Tree is sacred to the Hindus and Buddhists. Flower is an essential item of *Saraswati Puja.*

BAUHINIA VAHLII WT. & ARN. (CAESALPINIACEAE)

Syn : *Phanera vahlii* Benth.

Vernacular names: Ben: Sehari; **Lod** : Jom-Iar; **San:** Sihari-chop.

Traditional use: *TRIBES OF TEHRI-GARHWAL* : (i) *Fruit:* aphrodisiac, (ii) *Seed:* tonic and vermifuge; *TRIBES OF BASTAR* : (i) *Seed:* tonic; *SANTAL:* (i) *Plant:* in dysentery, stomachache, (ii) *Fruit:* to treat antifertility of women.

Phytography : Huge climber with many tendrils; branch lets hairy; leaves alternate, petiolate, simple, 2-cleft, cleavage goes down a quarter to one-third way from the apex, 7. 5-45. 0 cm long; racemes terminal, subcorymbose; flowers bracteate, 2. 5 cm long; pods nearly 45 by 5 cm, rusty-downy, 7-to 12-seeded.

Distribution: Foot of central and eastern Himalaya, ascending up to 800 m, Bihar, Madhya Pradesh, Maharashtra and Karnataka.

CAREYA ARBÓREA ROXB. (LECYTHIDACEAE)

English name: Tummy wood.

Sanskrit name: Kumbhi.

Vernacular names: Ben and **Hin** : Kumbhi; **Guj** : Kumbi; **Kan** : Kaval, Doddala, Asanda; **Lod** : Kumbi-daru, Kumbhi; **Mal:** Alam, Pelu; **Mun** : Asanda-daru, Kumbhir; **Sad:** Kumbi; **San:** Khubati; **Tam:** Ayma; **Tel:** Araya, Duddipa.

Trade names: Kumbhi, Kumbi.

Traditional use: *LODHA:* (i) *Root-paste:* in body pain, (ii) *Root-bark decoction* (with long pepper) : in fever, (iii) *Stem-bark powder* (paste with honey) : to children in cold and cough; *SANTAL* : *Stem-bark:* (paste with margosa) : in leucoderma

Phytography : Medium-sized tree with large ovate, ovate-oblong leaves clustered at the end of the branchlets, old le_ves often red/purple; flowers large, white and pink, in dense spikes, fruits large globose green, crowded with calyx tube, deciduous.

Phenology: *Flowering:* March-May; *Fruiting:* July.

Distribution : Sub-Himalayan tract occu-rring throughout India up to an elevation of 1700 m.

Chemical contents: *Bark:* lupeol, betulin; *Leaf:* ellagic acid, hexacosanol, quercetin, â-sitosterol, â-spinasterol taraxerol and its OAc, valoneic acid, careaborin, â-amyrin; *Seed:* á-spinasterol, á-spinasterone, baringtogenol-C, careyagenol-E.

Remarks: Only plant named by William Roxburgh in honour of William Carey. Lodhas use fresh stem bark decoction for washing septic wounds of cattle, and keep a dry fruit in a room as snake repellant. Oraons use powdered stem, root and leaf for poisoning fish.

CATHARANTHUS ROSEUS (L.) G. DON (APOCYNACEAE)

Syn: *Lochnera rosea* (L.) Spach, *Vinca rosea* L.

English names: Madagascar periwinkle, Old maid, Red periwinkle.

Vernacular names: Ben: Nayantara; **Hin** : Sada sawagon; **Lad:** Swet chandu; **Mal:** Ushamalari; **Mar:** Sadaphul; **Ori** : Ainskati; **Pun:** Rattanjot; **Tam:** Sudukadu Mallikai; **Tel:** Billaganneru. -

Trade name: Nayantara.

Traditional use: *BODO:* (i) *Plant:* in cancer, diabetes, (ii) *Leaf:* in menorrhagia; *LODHA* : (i) *Root-paste:* in septic wounds, (ii) *Root-decoction* (with paste of long peppers) : in fever, (iii) *Leaf-juice:* in blood dysentery, (iv) *Leaf-decoction:* to babies in gripping pain; *SANTAL* : (i) *Latex:* in scabies, (ii) *Seed-powder* (with decoction of black pepper) : in epilepsy; *ETHNIC COMMUNITIES OF EAST GODAVARI DISTRICT: Root:* in cancerous wounds.

Modern use: *Plant-extract:* antimitotic; *Root* (alkaloids) : in cancer, and as emetic, hypotensive, sedative and antiviral.

Phytography : A small herb or subshrub, up to 75 cm high; leaves elliptic-ovate to oblong, 4-10 by 2-4 cm, glabrous to puberulous, base acute or cuneate, apex obtusely apiculate, lateral nerves 10-12 pairs, petiole 1. 0-1. 5 cm; flowers in axillary or terminal cymes; solitary or paired, shortly pedicellate, pink or white or white with pink or yellow ring in orifice region; mericarps 3-4 by 0. 3 cm, puberulous.

Phenology: *Flowering* and *Fruiting:* throughout the year.

Distribution: A native of West Indies; commonly grown in gardens throughout India;

Bangladesh and Pakistan.

Ecology and cultivation: Plains from the coasts, in wastelands, fallow fields, less on the hills 800-1400 m, also widely cultivated.

Chemical contents : *Root-bark:* vincaline I & II; *Root:* vinblastine or vinleukoblastine (VLB), vincristine or vinleurocristine (VCR), ursolic acid, oleanolic acid, ajmalicine, alstonine; *Stem:* vinca rodine, vincoline, vinamidine, leurocolombine, vincathicine, vincubine; *Leaf:* leurosine, vindoline, catharanthine, lochnerine, tetrahydroalstonine, roseoside, essential oil; *Seed:* vincedine, vincedicine, tabersonine.

CURCUMA LONGA L. (ZINGIBERACEAE)

Syn : *Curcuma domestica* Val.

English name: Turmeric.

Sanskrit name: Haridra.

Vernacular names: Asm : Holodhi; **Ben:** Halud; **Guj** : Halada; **Hin** : Haldi; **Kan** : Arisina; **Kon** : Holldi, Ghor hollad; **Mal:** Manjella-kua; **Mar:** Halede; **Mun** : Hatu sasang, Sasang; **Orn:** Balka; **Ori** : Haladi; **Sad:** Haldi; **San:** Oerel sasan; **Tam:** Manjal; **Tel:** Pasupu.

Trade name: Haldi.

Traditional use: *ETHNIC COMMUNITIES OF ARUNACHAL PRADESH AND ASSAM: Rhizome:* in migrain; *SANTALS* : (i) *Rhizome:* in hazy vision, inflammation of eye, night blindness, subnormal temperature after fever, spleen consumption, *Basli rog* (pain similar to rheumatism), rheumatism due to draught, lock-jaw, *Rosbi* (stealth convulsions with indistinct speech), chronic scabies, sores and curbuncles, infantile atrophy, indigestion, prolapsus ani and fistula ani, bronchitis, cough and cold, puerperal fever; (ii) *Extract of Rhizome:* in rhagades; (iii) *Bulb:* in drying up of lactation; (iv) *Flower:* in cholera, sores in throat, syphilis; (v) *Dried Flower:* in icterus; *ETHNIC COMMUNITIES OF RANCHI* and *HAZARIBAGH (Bihar)* : (i) *Leaf:* in cold, fever, pneumonia; *GARHWALI: Rhizome:* in pimples and feckles on face, wounds, leprosy; *KUMAONI* : *Rhizome:* in cough, insect stings, wounds; *ETHNIC COMMUNITIES OF KURUKSHETRA* (Haryana) : *Rhizome:* in body pain, headache; *TRIBES OF ARAKU VALLEY* (Andhra Pradesh) : *Rhizome:* as anthelmintic..

RIGVEDA : *Rhizome:* improves body complexion and apetite; *YAJURVEDA* : *Rhizome:* is a blood-purifier, improves body complexion; *CHARAKA SAMHITA* : laxative, useful in leprosyand against contaminuos microbes; *SUSHRUTA SAMHITA* : digestive; *AYURVEDA* : *Rhizome:* effective against bacterial infection, skin diseases, intestinal worms, liver complaints, stammering, filaria, asthma, sprain, boils, wounds, conjuctivitis, thirst due to phlegm, allergic reactions, against leeches, minor ingredient of a drug for malarial fever.

SIDDHA : *Rhizome:* ingredient of *Kappu mancal, Manchal.*

UNANI : ingredient of 'Majnoor-e-falsfa', useful in gastrointestinal complaints; *Powder of rhizome:* used as antifertility agent.

Modern use: *Rhizome:* ingredient of 'Geriforte'-effective in senile pruritis, *Vitafix*-useful in premature ejaculation, insect repellent against houseflies, insecticide, antifungal; *EtOH* (50%) *extract of rhizome:* antiprotozoal, spasmolytic, hypotensive, Central Nervous System depressant; daily consumption of 1 gm raw rhizome helps to fight decaying metabolism and thus prevents cancer; *Essential oil from rhizome:* anti-arthritic, antifungal,. anti-inflammatory, antibacterial.

Phytography : Herb with large ovoid rootstock, sessile tubers thick, cylindric, bright yellow inside; petiole 60 cm long, leav. es green, 30-45 cm by 10-20 cm; peduncle 15 cm or more long, hidden by sheathing petiole, spikes 10-15 cm, about 5 cm in diameter; bracts pale green, ovate, about 3. 7 cm long, those of the coma pale pink; flowers yellow, as long as the bracts.

Phenology: *Flowering:* Autumn.

Distribution: Indigenous to Paresnath (Bihar); widely cultivated in West Bengal and other parts of India; Bangladesh, Sri Lanka.

Ecology and cultivation: Tropical plant; cultivated throughout the tropics. Chemical contents: *Essential oil from rhizome:* curcumin.

Remarks: In Hawaii, rhizome is used against growth of nostrils, for cleaning blood and as gargle; green rhizome is given for whooping and other coughs. In Sri Lanka, Rhizome paste is used in skeletal fracture. Extensive research is being carried out on the nutritional and medicinal value of this plant.

COSTUS SPECIOSUS (KOENING EX RETZ.) J. E. SMITH (ZINGIBERACEAE)

Syn : *Banksea speciosa* J. Koening

Sanskrit names: Canda, Kemuka.

Vernacular names: Ben: Keu; **Hin** : Kebu, Keyu, Kusi; **Kan** : Chengaivakoshtu; **Mal:** Cannakilannu, Cannakkuvva, Narumeanna; **Mar:** Penva, Pushkarmula; **Tam:** Kostam, Kuiravam, Kottam; **Tel:** Chengaivakohtu.

Trade name: Keyu.

Traditional use: *Rhizome:* bitter, astringent, acrid, cooling, purgative, aphrodisiac, anthelmintic, depurative, febrifuge, expectorant and tonic, also beneficial in asthma, anaemia, bronchitis, leprosy, flatulence, constipation, fever, skin diseases and inflammation.

Modern use: in carcino-genic tumours.

Phytography : Succulent perennial herb with long leafy spirally twisted stems, 2-3 m high and horizontal rhizomes; leaves simple, spirally arranged, ob-lanceolate or oblong, glabrous above, silky pubescent beneath with broad leaf sheaths; flowers white, large, scented, in large terminal spikes; bracts bright red; fruits globose/ovoid capsules; seeds obovoid or semi-globose.

Phenology: *Flowering:* September-October; inflorescence globose of closely packed bracts.

Distribution: Throughout India; Pakistan and Bangladesh-in moist localities and in wastelands.

Ecology and cultivation: Hills above 800 m; moist places and wastelands also.

Chemical content: *Root:* rich in starch.

DATURA METEL L. (SOLANACEAE)

Syn : *Datura alba* Nees, *D. fastuosa* L. var *alba* C. B. Clarke

English name: Hindu datura.

Sanskrit name: Dhustura.

Vernacular names :Ben: Dhutra, Dhatura; **Hin** : Sadahdhatura; **Tam:** Vellum mattai. **Trade name:** Dhutra.

Traditional use: *FOLKS OF PURULIA (West Bengal* and *Rajasthan: Seed:* for treatment of leprosy; *FOLKS OF RAJASTHAN: Leaf:* in guinea-worms; *Other uses of seed, leaf* and *root:* in insanity, fever with catarrhal and cerebral complications, diarrhoea, skin diseases and antideptic. It is narcotic, acrid, anodyne, antispasmodic, intoxicating, emetic and useful in asthma; *Root:* used for treatment of bites from rabbits; *Poultice made of leaf:* used for epilepsy, ophthalmodynia, otalgia, lumbago, sciatica, neuralgia, mumps and painful swelling.

Modern use: *Seed:* aphrodisiac, narcotic and antispasmodic and useful in dontalgia, otalgia, gastropathy and skin diseases and for treatment of dandruff and lice; *EtOH* (50%) *extract of plant:* anticancer, anthelmintic, spasmogenic and blood pressure depressant;*Aquous extract of plant:* nematicidal; *Leaf extract:* antiviral; *EtOH extract of leaf* and *aquous extract of fruit:* anticholinergic.

Phytography : Coarse annual herb, may be 2 m tall, stem scented; leaf alternate, petiolate, simple; flowers axillary, peduncled, white or nearly so, 17. 5 cm long and may be 12. 5 cm in diameter across the mouth; capsules subglobose, 3 cm in diameter, equally spinous on all sides.

Phenology: *Flowering:* throughout the year; *Fruiting:* with blunt spines.

Distribution: Throughout India; occasionally grown in gardens.

Ecology and Cultivation: Hills up to 1500 m, occasionally in the plains even to the coast; wild.

Chemical contents: *Root:* alkaloids, tropane derivatives; *Stem:* hyoscine, hyoscyamine, Leaf: hyoscine, hyoscyamine, micotianamine; *Fruit (pericarp)* :

alkaloids, â-sitosterol, triterpene, daturaolone, daturadiol; *Seed:* hyosane, hyoscyamine, daturaolone, fastusic acid; *Seed-oil:* â-Me-sterols.

DIOSPYROS PEREGRINA (GAERTN.) GURKE (EBENACEAE)

Syn : *Diospyros embryoteris* Pers., *D malabarica* (Oeser.) Kost.

English names: Gaub Persimmon, Wild Mangostein.

Sanskrit names: Kalaskardha, Krishnasara, Tinduka.

Vernacular names: Ben and **Hin** : Gab, Kata Gab; **Kan** : Holetupari; **Mal:** Panachi; **Mar:** Tender; **Ori** : Dhusarokendu, Kendu; **San:** Makar kenda; **Tam:** Katlati, Tumbi; **Tel** : Tinduki.

Traditional use: *SANTAL* : (i) *Root:* in gravel; (ii) *Bark:* in cholera; (iii) *Fruit:* in dysentery and menorrhagia; *TRIBES OF ABUJH-MARH RESERVE AREA* (Madhya Pradesh) : *Fruit:* in dysentery and as tonic; *TRIBES OF BASTAR* (Madhya Pradesh) : *Fruit:* in blister in mouth, diarrhoea.

HARIT SAMHITA : *Bark:* in gastro-enteritis; *BAGBHATTA* : *Juice of unripe fruit:* in restoring normal skin colour after burn; *BHABAPRAKASA* : *Aqueous extract of green fruit:* in healing burn-wound; *BANGASENA* : *Powder of dried fruit with honey:* licking is beneficial in hiccup in children.

AYURVEDA : (i) *Bark extract:* in chronic dysentery; (ii) *Aqueous extract of green fruit:* in menorrhagia, excessive salivation.

Modern Use: *EtOH* (50%) *extract of stem* and *leaf:* anticancer, diuretic; *EtOH* (50%) *extract of stem bark:* antiprotozoal, antiviral, hypoglycaemic.

Phytography : Middle-sized, profusely branched tree; stem and branches black, branchlets glabrous; leaves alternate, petioles ±0. 6 to ±0. 8 cm long, lamina thick, leathery, oblong, veines slightly elevated above; male flowers in few or many-flowered short cymes, flowers tubular, 0. 8 cm long, lobed, calyx black, silky; female flowers solitary or few together, subsessile or cymose, larger than male flowers, ovary 8-celled; fruits usually solitary, subglobose, 2. 5-5. 0 cm in diameter, brick-coloured when young, yellowish when mature, persistent calyx lobed, accrescent 4-to 8 -seeded.

Phenology: *Flowering* and *Fruiting:* Summer to rainy season, fruits take 4-5 months to mature.

Distribution Throughout India; Bangladesh, Malaysia and other South-East Asian countries, also in Australia.

Ecology and cultivation: Throughout India, abundant in Bengal; cultivated near habitational sites; occasionally found as ferals; Sri Lanka.

Chemical contents: *Root:* glycerides; *Bark:* myricyle alcohol, saponin, triterpenes; *Stem:* â-sitosterol, á leuconanthocyanin; *Leaf:* triterpenes; *Fruit pulp:* alkenes, triterpenes; *Seed:* betulinic acid, â-amyrin, fatty oil, unsaponified matter.

Adulterants: Often it is confused with *Garcinia mangostana* and *Strychnos nux-vomica.* **Remarks:** Santals use bark in treatment of rinderpest.

Rural people of North Bengal and Bangladesh consume the leaves as vegetable. Fruits are eaten by Bhoxas, Lodhas, Monpas, Santals and Bengalees.

Tribes of Bastar consume the seeds.

Boatmen rub the fruit-juice on the undersurface of boats to protect the wood from rotting, and fishermen use the same in their fishing net for the same purpose.

DOLICHOS BIFLORUS L. (FABACEAE)

Syn : *Dolichos uniflorus* Lam., *Glycine uniflora* Dalz.

English name: Horsegram.

Sanskrit name: Kulattha.

Vernacular names: Ben: Kurti-kalai; **Hin** and **Mar:** Kutthi; **Kan** : Hurali; **Mal:** Muthiva; **Man:** Nagakrijon; **Mun** : Kurthi; **Orn** : Anrsga; **Sad:** Kurthi; **San:** Horec; **Tam:** Kollu; **Tel:** Ulavalu.

Traditional use: *SANTAL* : (i) *plant:* dysuria, sores, tumours; (ii) *leaf:* in burns; (iii) *seed:* **in** adenitis, *fistula ani,* intercostal neuralgia, pleurisy, pneumonia, *prolapsus ani; MUNOA* : *aqueous extract of seed:* to women after childbirth; *IRULA, KOTA, TOOA* (Nilgiri) : *seed:* in menstrual complaints; *RURAL FOLKS: Aqueous extract of seed:* in urinary troubles and kidney stone.

CHARAKA SAMHITA : *seed:* useful in piles, hiccup, abdominal lump, bronchial asthma, in causing and regulating perspiration; *SUSHRUTA SAMHITA. seed powder:* useful in stopping excessive perspiration; *BAGBHATTA: seed:* useful in spermatocalcali *(Shukrashman); CHAKRADATTA* : *decoction of seed:* beneficial in urticaria; *RAJANIGHANTU* : beneficial in piles, colic, epistasis, flatulence, ophthalmia, ulcer.

AYURVEDA : *decoction of seed:* useful in leucorrhoea, menstrual troubles, bleeding during pregnancy, colic caused by wind, piles, rheumatism, heamorrhagic disease, intestinal worms; *seed powder:* antidiaphoretic; *seed* (in combination with milk) : work as anthelmintic, soup prepared from seeds is beneficial in enlarged liver and spleen.

SIDDHA : *seed:* used in preparing a medicine named *Kollu.*

Modern use: *Plant extract:* radiolabel reagent in ABa blood grouping of human hair; *EtOH* (50%) *extract of Seed:* spasmolytic.

Phytography : Annual herb, trailing or suberect, branched; leaves alternate, stipulate, trifoliate, leaflets membranous, ovate, ±2. 5-5. 0 cm long, young ones finely pilose; flowers axillary, may be more than one together but without a common peduncle, papilionaceous, usually yellow-may be white, ±1. 25-1. 8

cm long; pods ±3. 7-5. 0 cm by 0. 6-0. 8 cm, recurved, tipped with a persistent style; seeds 5-6 per pod, ellipsoid, flattened.

Phenology: *Flowering:* August-November; *Fruiting:* September-December.

Distribution: Widely distributed in India, ascending up to 1000 m in Sikkim; cultivated mainly in Andhra Pradesh, Tamil Nadu, Karnataka.

Ecology and cultivation: Mesophyte; wild and cultivated.

Chemical contents: *Stem* and *Leaf:* coumesterol, a lectin-like glycoproticin, psoraliding; *Leaf* (bacteria treated) : dolichin A and dolichin B; *Seed* : â-sitosterol, coumesterol, delbergiodin, genistein, 2-hydroxy-genistein, isoferreirin, keivitone, phaseollidin, pyranoside.

Adulterant: *Cassia abrus* L. is sometimes confused with this plant.

Remarks: Santals use the plant in treatment of *rinderpest* of domestic animals. Seeds are often consumed as pulse. Santals consider eating this pulse is good for patients of dysentery and leprosy, but they prohibit eating this by the patients of measles and small pox.

DILLENIA INDICA L. (DILLENIACEAE)

Syn : *Dillenia speciosa* Thunb.

English name: Dillenia.

Sanskrit names: Bhavya, Bharija.

Vernacular names: Asm : Chalita, Qutenga; **Ben:** Chalta; **Guj** : Karambel; **Hin** : Chalta; **Kan** :Betta kanijala; **Mar:** Mota karmal; **Mal:** Chalita, Punna; **Man:** Heigri; **Ori** : Qu, Uvu; **San:** Korbhatta; **Tam** and **Tel:** Uva.

Trade name: Chalta.

Traditional use: *MANIPURI* : *Fruit decoction:* for curing dandruff and checking falling of hairs; *MIKIR* (Assam) : *Fruit:* eat to combat weakness; *TRIBES OFTEJPUR* (Assam) : *Plant:* in fever; *TRIBES OF TIRAP* (Arunachal Pradesh) : *Leaf:* in dysentery; *SANTAL* : (i) *Root:* as prophylactic at the cholera season, an ingredient of a medicine for burning sensation in the chest; (ii) *Stem-bark:* component of medicine for sores caused by mercury poisoning, chronic progredient sores and carbuncle, and as a prophylactic at the cholera season; (iii) *Mucilage:* on wounds of burns; *TRIBES OF ABUJH MARH RESERVE AREA* (Madhya Pradesh) : *Fruit:* as tonic; *TRIBES OF EAST GODAVARI* (Andhra Pradesh) : *Fleshy calyx:* in stomach disorders.

YAJURVEDA : an important plant; *UPAVARHANA SAMHITA* : the plant is aphrodisiac and prpmotes virility; *CHARAKA SAMHITA* : the fruit is sweet, acidic, astringent, removes bile, phlegm, fetid and flatulence; *SUSHRUTA SAMHITA* : fruit cardiotonic, tasteful, astringent, acidic, removes bile, phlegm, fetid and flatulence; *RAJANIGHANTU:* green fruit is acidic, pungent, hot, removes wind, phlegm, but the ripe fruit is sweet, sour, appetising and beneficial in colic associated with mucous; *MATSYA PURANA* : decoction of this plant can be used as universal antidote for poison; *AGNI PURANA* : spraying water, containing stem extract, on and around the wound caused by spider bite helps in removing the poison.

AYURVEDA: (i) *Root (bark extrac_:* in food poisoning; (ii) *Root-bark(paste)* : along with leaf-paste applied externally in sprains; (iii) *Young bark* and *Leaf:* astringent; (iv) *Fruit-juice* : mixed with sugar and water serves as a cooling beverage in fever, fit, and as a cough syrup; (v) *Ripe fruit-juice:* removes flatulence, increases quantity of semen, galactogogue, combats weakness, external application helps supuration of boil, and checks loss of hair.

Modern use: *Leaf* (50% *EtOH extract)* : shows antiamphetamine activity; *Seed-extract:* antimicrobial; *Seed-oil:* antifungal, and its unsaponifiable matter antibacterial.

Phytography : Evergreen, round-headed tree, 9-42. 5 m high; branchlets tomentose, bark cinnamomum-like; leaf alternate, simple, fascicled at the apices of branches, petiole 3. 7 cm long, lamina 20-25 cm by 5-10 cm, oblong-Ianceolate, closely set parallel veins from midrib, upper surface glabrous, hairs present on the lower surface, especially on veins; flower terminal or leaf-opposed, solitary, white, 15 cm in diameter, sepals thick; fruit globose with accrescent calyx, 12. 5-15 cm in diameter, green when young, yellowish and sweet-scented when ripe; seeds many, compressed, embedded in hairy cells.

Phenology: *Flowering:* May-June; *Fruiting:* July-August. -ripens in November-December.

Distribution: Sub-Himalayan tract from Garhwal to Assam, Arunachal Pradesh, Manipur, Tripura, West Bengal, Orissa, Bihar, Central and South India; Nepal, Bangladesh, Sri Lanka.

Ecology and cultivation: Plant of tropical forest; occasionally grown in gardens.

Chemical contents: *Stem-bark:* betulin, betulinaldehyde, betulic acid, flavonoids, dillentin, dihydroisorhamnetin, lupeol, myricetin, glucosides, B-sitosterol; *Wood:* betulinic acid, lupeol, â-sitosterol; *Leaf:* betulinic acid, cycloartenone, flavonoids, n-hentriacontanol, B-sitosterol; *Fruit:* an arabinogalactan, betulinic acid, â-sitosterol.

Remark: Green calyx is eaten in various forms of pickles.

DIOSCOREA BULBIFERA L. (DIOSCOREACEAE)

Syn : *Dioscorea crispata* Roxb., *D. pulchella* Roxb.. *D. sativa* Thunb. non L, *D. versicolor* Buch. Ham.

English names: Air yam, Potato yam, Air potato.

Sanskrit name: Varahi.

Vernacular names: Ben: Banalu, Kukuralu; **Hin** : Gaithi, Rataler, Pitalu; **Kan** : Heggenasu; **Man:** Ha; **Mar:** Manakundu, Karukarinda; **Mun** : Jo aru; **Tam:** Kodikulangu; **Tel:** Chedupaddu-dumpa; **San:** Bongo-sanga.

Traditional use: *TRIBES OF PURULIA* (West Bengal) : *Tuber:* in boils; *SANTAL* : (i) *Dried tuber (powdery:* as shampoo and on sores; (ii) *Plant:* against madness; *SIKKIMESE* : *Tuber:* in jaundice; *ETHNIC COMMUNITIES OF DEHRA DUN* AND *SIWALIK: Tuber:* in dysentery, piles; *DANG* (Gujarat) : *Tuber:* in abdominal pain, bone fracture.

Modern use: *Aerial parts* (50% *EtOH extract)* : diuretic; *Rhizome:* anorexiant.

Phytography : Climber, usually twining to the left; stem slender, green or purple, with 10-15 small crisped wings, tubers large, variable in form; leaves opposite and alternate, petioles 5-15 cm long, lamina cordate, very variable in size, attaining 35 cm in length, membranous, dark green, 7-9 costate; male spikes slender, almost capillary, 2. 5-10 cm long, panicled, flowers crowded or scattered, green or purplish; female spikes 10-25 cm long, pendulous; capsules 1. 6-2. 5 cm by 0. 8-1. 25 cm, membranous; seeds with broad basal wing.

Phenology: *Flowering:* August-September; *Fruiting:* November.

Distribution: Common in the outskirts of forests throughout India, ascending up to 2000 m in the hills; Bangladesh, Pakistan.

Ecology and cultivation: Plant of tropical climate, grows in the midst of scrub jungles, rare; wild and planted.

Chemical contents: *Tuber:* furanoid norditerpenes, norditerpene glucosides, diosbulbinoside D & F, diosbulbin B & D, a new dihydrophenanthrene, d-sorbitol; *Bulbil:* diosgenin.

Remarks: Tubers are eaten as vegetable by the ethnic communities of Meghalaya, Kameng district of Arunachal Pradesh, Purulia and Medinipur districts of West Bengal, Varanasi, Mirzapur districts and Kumaon area of Uttar Pradesh, Madhya Pradesh, Goa, Maharashtra, Ratan Mahal Hills (Gujarat), Rajasthan, Cannanore district of Kerala and Mikirs (Assam), Santals (West Bengal) and Tharus (Uttar Pradesh).

Boiled bulbils are eaten by Mikirs and Santals as vegetable.

ELETTARIA CARDAMOMUM (L.) MATON (ZINGIBERACEAE)

Syn : *Cardamum officinale* Salisb.; *(non-Ammomum cardamum* L. 1753); *Alpinia cardamum* Roxb.

English names: Cardomum, Lesser cardamum.

Sanskrit names: Ela, Trutih.

Vernacular names: Ben: Chhoto elach; **Guj** : Elachi; **Hin** : Chhoti elaichi;

Kan : Yellaki; **Mal:** Cittelum, Elam; **Mar:** Elachi veldodi; **Tam:** Elam; **Tel:** Yelakkayalu.

Trade name: Chhoti elaichi.

Traditional use: *MATSYA PURANA* : a constituent of an antivenom drug.

AYURVEDA : seeds abortifacient, alexiteric, aromatic, acrid, sweet, cooling, carminative, cardiac tonic, digestive, diuretic, expectorant, stimulant, and tonic, beneficial in asthma, bronchitis, strangury, haemorrhoids, renal and vesical calculi, halitosis, anorexia, dyspepsia, gastropathy and burning sensation.

SIDDHA : dried fruit, seed and stem-bark are used to prepare drugs cell 'Elam', 'Elarici'.

UNANI: preparations used as antidote to poison, astringent, exhilarant and in nausea.

Modern use: *Essential oil from seed:* antimicrobial; oil is used in several pharmaceutical preparations.

Phytography : Perennial leafy herb, 1. 5-3. 0 m high; rootstock thick, horizontal; leaves 30-65 cm by 5-10 cm, distichous, elliptic or elliptic-Ianceolate, glabrous above, softly pubescent below, acuminate at apex, narrowed or obtuse at base; flowers white, striped with violet, in elongated, flexuous, bracts, panicles arising from the rootstock; capsules oblong or subindehiscent, marked with fine vertical ribs; seeds black, arillate.

Phenology: *Flowering* and *Fruiting:* throughout the year, mainly in late autumn and winter.

Distribution: Found in rich, moist forests of the hilly tracts, up to 2000 m; commercially cultivated in Tamil Nadu, Andhra Pradesh, Karnataka, Gujarat.

Ecology and cultivation: Plant of tropical moist climate; wild and cultivated.

Chemical contents: Seed : essential oil, terpenoids.

Remark: Fruits and seeds are used as masticator.

EMBELIA RIBES BURM. F. (MYRSINACEAE)

Syn : *Embelia glandulifera* Wight, *Samara ribes* Kurz

English names: Embelia, Embelia fruit.

Sanskrit names: Jantughna, Krimighna, Krimiripu, Vella, Vidanga.

Vernacular names: Ben: Biranga; **Guj** : Vaivarang, Vavading; **Hin** : Baberang, Vayvidang; **Kan** : Vayuvilanga; **Mar:** Vaivarang, Vavadinga; **Mal:** Vizhal; **Pun:** Baburung; **Tam** and **Tel:** Vayuvilanga.

Traditional use: *GARHWALI* and *TRIBES OF NORTH-EAST INDIA: Seed:*

in skin diseases, ringworms, leprosy; *ETHNIC COMMUNITIES OF KAMRUP* (Assam) : *Fruit:* in stomach complaints.

MATSYA PURANA : important medicinal plant; *AGNI PURANA* : beneficial for gastroenteritis, cirrhosis of liver, oedema, skin diseases including leprosy and effective in killing worms in alimentary canal; *VIJACINTAMANITANTRA:* consumption of powdered fruit along with fruits of *Emblica officinalis,* honey and sesame-oil improves quality of sperms; *BHAVAPRAKASHA:* it is pungent, removes morbidity, improves blood circulation, stimulates appetite, acts against phlegm, makes the body light, kills worms of all types; *RAJANIGHANTU:* it is pungent, hot, light, enhances balance between wind and phlegm, beneficial in anorexia and improves digestive power.

AYURVEDA : (a) *Root:* acrid, astringent, useful in colic, dyspepsia, flatulence, odontalgia, stomach pain and increases exothermic metabolism; (b) *Leaf:* astringent, demulcent, depurative, thermogenic, useful in skin diseases including leprosy; (c) *Fruit:* acrid, alexeteric, alterant, anodyne, anthelmintic, astringent, bitter, brain tonic, carminative, contraceptive, depurative, digestive, diuretic, febrifuge, laxative, rejuvenating, stimulant, tonic, vulnerary, and useful in amnetia, asthma, colic, constipation, cardiopathy, dental caries, dyspepsia, dyspnoea, fever, flatulence, general debility, hemicramia, odontalgia, psychopathy, respiratory troubles and ring-worms; (d) *Seed:* a constituent of *Vidangadi Yoga,* an antifertility drug.

SIDDHA : dried fruits are used to prepare the drug *Vaivitankam.*

Modern use : *Plant:* cures abdominal tumours, and aenemeas, cystic tumours, pyorrhoea, useful against tape-worms; *EtOH extract of plant:* slightly active against *Ecoli;* one of the constituents of 'Gasex', and some oral contraceptives; *Fruit:* cures dental, oral, throat troubles except cancer of lips and ptyslism, constituent of some quick aboriticide; *Aqueous extract of fruit:* pronounced antifertility activity, anthelmintic against earthworms;*Fruit-powder:* expels tapeworms within 6-24 hours, if taken with curd in empty stomach, effective against giardia; *Seed:* antibiotic, anthelmintic, antituberculosis, alterative and stimulative.

Phytography : Large scandent shrub; branches long, slender, flexible, bark with many lenticels; leaves simple, alternate, petioles ±0. 8 cm, lamina elliptic, leathery, glabrous, shining above, silvery beneath, glandular pits present on the lower surface near the midrib; racemes axillary and terminal, laxly panicled; flowers white, may be greenish, ±0. 2 cm long; berries dull red to black, globular, small, 1-or 2-seeded; seeds globose, hollowed at the base, white spotted, albuminous.

Phenology: *Flowering:* peak in March-April; *Fruiting:* August.

Distribution: Throughout India up to 1750 m in hilly regions; common in lower hills; Sri Lanka, Malaya.

Ecology and cultivation: Grows in shola border, thickets; wild.

Chemical contents: *Fruit:* embelin.

Remark: Ethnic communities of Cannanore (Kerala) make bowstring with the bark.

ECLIPTA ALBA (L.) ROXB. (ASTERACEAE)

Syn : *Eclipta prostrata* (L.) Hassk.

English name: Trailing eclipta.

Sanskrit names: Bhringa, Bhringaraja, Kesaraja, Kayyonni, Markava, Tekarajah. **Vernacular names: Asm** : Kehoraji; **Ben:** Bhringaraj, Keshurti, Kesuria, Keshurey; **Guj** : Bhengra; **Hin** : Babri, Bhangra, Mocakand, Safed bhannra; **Kan** : Garga; **Mal** : Kannunni, Kaiyanni, Kayyonni; **Man:** Oochisumbal; **Mar:** Maka; **Mun** : Bhengaj, Piri kesari; **Om** : Bhengraj; **Ori** :Kesarda; **Sad:** Bhengrait; **San:** Banda-kansa; **Tam:** Garuga, Kaikesi, Karipan, Kayyantakara; **Tel:** Galagara, Guntagalyeru.

Trade name: Kesuth

Traditional use: *GARO: Leaf:* in gastric troubles, hepatic disorders; *MANIPURI* : (i) *Stem-decoction:* in liver enlargement; (ii) *Leaf-extract:* in fever and cough; *TOTO:* (i) *Whole plant:* in hepatic problems, spleen troubles; (ii) *Root:* in ulcers and wounds; (iii) *Leaf:* as antidote to scorpion sting; *ETHNIC COMMUNITIES OF ORISSA:* (i) *Plant:* in itching; (ii) *Leaf:* in conjunctivitis and other eye problems, in promoting hairgrowth; *SANTAL* : (i) *Plant-decoction with paste of black pepper:* in fever; (ii) *Leaf-juice:* on wounds; *ETHNIC COMMUNITIES OF BIHAR:* (i) *Plant:* against antifertility, (ii) *Root:* as antidote to snake bite; (iii) *Leaf:* in malaria and other fevers; *ETHNIC COMMUNITIES OF ARAKU VALLEY* (Madhya Pradesh) : *Leaf:* in conjunctivitis, eye troubles; *IRULAR: Leaf:* in jaundice; *TRIBAL SOCIETIES OF ANAIKATTY HILLS* (Tamil Nadu) : *Flower bud:* in fever, headache; *ETHNIC COMMUNITIES OF SALSETTE ISLAND: Leaf:* as cooling; *TRIBAL SOCIETIES OF SAURASHTRA* (Gujarat) : *Whole Plant:* in asthma, bronchitis, leucoderma; *TRIBAL SOCIETIES OF EASTERN RAJASTHAN: Leaf:* in sores, ulcers, wounds, spleen disorders; *TRIBES OF KURUKSHETRA* (Haryana) : *Leaf:* as antiseptic; *GARHWALI:* (i) *Whole plant:* in jaundice, spleen disorders; (ii) *Leaf:* in leucoderma, skin diseases; *KOL* : *Leaf:* in malaria; *TRIBES OF BASTAR* (Madhya Pradesh) : *Whole plant:* in liver complaints; *TRIBES OF CHHINDWARA* (Madhya Pradesh) : *Leaf:* for promoting hair growth; *TRIBES OF SAGAR* (Madhya Pradesh) : *Plant:* in toothache, headache, gland swelling, elephantiasis.

ATHARVAVEDA : it affects intelligence and memory, cures bile *(pitta)* disorders, prevents graying and falling of hairs.

BHAVAPRAKASHA : cures problems caused by phlegm and wind, beneficial for hair, skin, teeth and eyes, removes worms, and also effective in jaundice and oedema; *RAJANIGHANTU:* beneficial for hairs, eyes, oedema and phlegm; *KAIYADEVANIGHANTU* : it removes the problems caused by phlegm and wind and worms, beneficial for hair, teeth, skin, cures cough, jaundice and oedema; *NIGHANTURATNAKARAM:* in addition to the above qualities, this plant invigorates sex; *VAIDYAMANORAMA* : drinking juice of the plant strengthens the body and secures the foetus in womb.

AYURVEDA : cures headache, migraine; leaves are beneficial for hairs, they remove lice, blacken skin, cure pyorrhoea, chronic dysentery, oedema, nervous weakness, jaundice, anorexia, gum troubles and remove intestinal worms.

Modern use: *Herb:* in skin diseases; *Gum resin* (from herb) : anticancerous against *Ehrlich ascites carcinoma; Plant(50% EtOH extract)*: antiviral, spasmogenic; *Plant (aqueous extract)* : ovicidal against *Sitotroga cerealella* eggs, nematicidal, haemostatic, beneficial in body inflammation, protective against hepatotoxic action of carbon tetrachloride in female guineapigs; *Plant* (powder) : curative of infective hepatitis, jaundice and viral hepiltitis; *Leaf(aqueous* extract) : myocardial depressant, hypotensive; *Leaf-juice:* cures shoulder pain caused by heavy load.

Phytography : Erect or prostrate diffused annual herb with roots at each node; leaves opposite, sessile, oblong-lanceolate, ±2. 5-1 0 cm long, very variable in form and width; heads subglobose, ±1. 25 cm broad; flowers white and compressed.

Phenology: *Flowering* and *Fruiting:* throughout the year, peak period-August--February.

Distribution: Throughout India, ascending up to 2000 m; Bangladesh and Pakistan.

Ecology and cultivation: Common on damp wastelands, low waterlogged areas, roadsides, grassy humid localities, prefers warm climate; wild.

Chemical contents: *Leaf:* stigmasterol, a-terthienyl methanol, wedelolactone, de-Me-wedelolactone, small amount of 2-formyl-terthienyl.

Adulterants: In Sanskrit literature, three types of *Bhringaraja* have been mentioned-white-flowered *(E. alba)*, yellow-flowered *(Wedelia calandulacea)* and blue--flowered (not yet identified).

Remarks: Tribals use juice of leaves for tattooing purpose.

EMBLICA OFFICINALIS GAERTN. (EUPHORBIACEAE)

Read: *Phyllanthus emblica* L.

English name: Emblica myrobalan.

Sanskrit names: Adiphala, Amlaka, Amritaphala, Dhatri, Hatha, Nellikka.

Vernacular names: Asm : Amluki; **Ben:** Amla, Amlaki; **Guj** : Amali; **Hin** : Amla, Aon, Aonala; **Kan** : Amalaka; **Mal:** Amalakam, Nelli; **Man:** Heikru; **Mar:** Anvala; **Mun** : Meral daru; **Orn** : Amra; **Ori** : Amla; **Pun:** Ambli, Ambuli; **Sad:** Aonra; **San:** Aohal; **Tam:** Nelli, Toppunelli; **Tel:** Amlakamu, Usirika.

Trade name: Amla, Amlaki.

Traditional use: *ETHNIC COMMUNITIES OF SAGAR DISTRICT* (Madhya Pradesh) : *Fruit:* antiemitic, used in fever, indigestion; *ETHNIC COMMUNIT/ES OF DEHRA DUN* and *SIWALIK DISTRICTS* (Uttar Pradesh) : *Fruit:* in bronchitis, indigestion; *Seed:* in asthma; *DANG* (Gujarat) : *Bark:* on burn, wounds, stomach complaint; *IRULAR* (Tamil Nadu) : *Leaf:* against cold; *BIRHoRE(West* Bengal) : *Fruit:* in constipation, headache, liver complaint, madness; *THANES* (Uttar Pradesh) : *Fruit:* in constipation; *ETHNIC COMMUNIT/ES OF GARHWAL* : *Fruit:* laxative, cooling, in diabetes, dysentery, and as diuretic; *ETHNIC* COMMUNIES *OF TIRAP* (Arunachal Pradesh) : *Fruit:* in diabetes; *NAGA: Fruit:* in eye complaint; *KHASI* and *JAINTIA* : *Fruit:* in eye complaint; *TRIBES OF MIRZA PUR DISTRICT* (Uttar Pradesh) : *Fruit:* in eye complaint; *TRIBES OF HAZARIBAGH DISTRICT* (Bihar) : *Fruit:* used to revive taste; *KOL* (Uttar Pradesh) : *Fruit:* on scorpion sting; *ETHNIC COMMUNITIES OF MAYURBHANJ* (Orissa) : *Fruit:* against thirst; *ORAON* : (i) *Fruit:* in cough; (ii) *Juice of fresh fruit* and (ii) *Infusion of seed:* in inflammation of eyes; (iv) *Crushed fruit* with fruit of *Terminalia citrin* a and *Terminalia belerica* macerated in a tumbler of water in the evening: a very good stomachic and tonic; *MANIPURI:* (i) *Boiled extract of leaf:* in controlling high blood sugar; (ij) *Fruit:* in constipation, bleeding gum, piles, blood diseases and also as brain and nerve tonic; *SANTAL:* (i) *Leaf:* in anaemia, diarrhoea, dysentery, fever, gravel, sores *(agya ghao, rokoc ghao);* (ii) *Stem-bark:* in cholera, profuse diarrhoea *(haga sitka),* fistula, sores *(bonga khoda, nason ghao, pachiari ghao, palania ghao);* (iii) *Powder of male inflorescence:* in nasal haemorrhage; (iv) *Infusion of green fruit:* in gripe; (v) *Ripe fruit:* in cystitis and diarrhoea.

RAJAN/GHANTU: it is acidic *(amla),* astringent *(kashaya), pleasant(madhura),* cooling and light, beneficial in burning sensation caused by deranged bile, vomiting, oedema and is rejuvenating; the fruit is appetising, antiemetic and removes fatigue, useful in constipation and flatulence.

AYURVEOA : Fruit is useful in acidity, urinary trouble, hiccup, vomiting, leucorrhoea, biliary colic, urticaria, conjunctivitis and dysentery.

SIOOHA : Root-bark, fruit-juice and dried fruit are used to prepare a medicine named *Nelli.*

Modern use: *Fruit:* pronounced expectorant, antioxidant, anticancerous; *EtOH* (50%) *extract of fruit:* antiviral, carminative, stomachic; *Aqueous extract of fruit:* increases cardiac glycogen level and decreases serum GOT, GPT and LDH in rats; *Fruit-juice:* (i) mixed with turmeric powder and honey: cures *diabetes insipidus;* (ii) in *ghee:* used for abdominal and glandular tumours; a constituent of the medicine *SG-1-Switradilepa* used against vitiligo, and of an antibiotic drug *Septilin.*

Phytography : Deciduous tree with flaky bark, greenish, grey or red; leaves distichously closely set, bipinnate, dark green, leaflets linear-oblong; flowers densely fascicled, yellowish, unisexual, males on slender pedicels while females subsessile; fruits light green when young, yellowish when mature, globose, depressed, succulent, obscurely six-lobed, one-seeded; seed trigonous.

Phenology: *Flowering:* February-May; *Fruiting:* May onwards.

Distribution: Common in the mixed deciduous forests of India, ascending up to 1500 m, often cultivated in gardens and homeyards; Bangladesh, Pakistan.
Ecology and cultivation: Plant of tropical climate; predominantly wild, cultivated in Uttar Pradesh, Madhya Pradesh.

Chemical contents: *Root:* ellagic acid, oleanolic acid, oleanolic aldehyde, lupeol; *Stem-bark:* lelucodel-phinidin, procyanidin, 3-0-gallated prodelphinidin and tannin; *Stem* and *Leaf:* lupeol, â-sitosterol; *Fruit:* vitamin C, carotene, riboflavine, D-glucose, D-fructose, myoinositol, nicotinic acid, D galacturoniaacid, phyllemblic acid, mucic acid, fatty acids, D-arabinosyl, D-xylosyl, L-rhamnosyl, D-glucosyl, D-mannosyl, D-galactosyl..

Remarks: Santals use bark in rinderpest, anthrax and convulsion of cattle. Fruits are eaten raw or as pickle and used to make ink. Wood is not attacked by insects.

EUPHORBIA TIRUCALLI L. (EUPHORBIACEAE)

English name : Milk bush, Indian tree spurge.

Sanskrit names : Shatala, Trikantaka.

Vernacular names: Ben: Ganderi, Lankasij, Latadoona; **Guj** : Thor dandalio; **Hin :** Konpol, Sehund; **Kan** : Bantakalli; **Mar:** Shera; **Tam:** Tirukalli, Kalli; **Tel:** Chemudu.

Trade name: Tirukalli.

Traditional use: *IRULAR: Latex:* in body pain, eczema, scabies; *ETHNIC COMMUNITIES OF CHAMPAKARAI and DHOOMANOOR* (Tamil Nadu) : *Latex:* on wounds; *NAYADI* : *Latex:* in rheumatism; *ETHNIC COMMUNITIES*

OF MADHYA PRADESH: Latex: in earache, rheumatism, warts; *ETHNIC COMMUNITIES OF CHHOTANAGPUR* : *Latex:* in earache.

BHAVAPRAKASHA: Itis pungent, bitter, helps digestion, beneficial in oedema, deranged phlegm, epistasis, deranged bile, constipation and dyscrasia.

AYURVEDA : *Root:* beneficial in colic; *Latex of stem and leaf:* cures cough, earache, emetic, laxative and rubefacient.

Modern use: *Stem-extract:* antifungal; *Aerial parts* (50% *EtOH extract)* : antiprotozoal.

Phytography : Erect tree, 3-6 m high, branches thin, cylindrical, spreading, scattered, clustered, whorled, latex extraordinarily abundant, sticky and acrid; leaves alternate, linear, caducous, petioles modified to phylloclade; involucres clustered in the forks of branches, inconspicuous, flowers shortly pedicelled, bracteoles numerous; cocci dark brown, velvety, compressed; seeds ovoid, smooth.

Phenology: *Flowering:* very scarce, mainly in June-July; *Fruiting:* July-October.

Distribution: Introduced from tropical Africa, naturalised in the drier parts of India; elsewhere largely cultivated as hedges and fuel plants.

Ecology and cultivation: Xerophytic.

Chemical contents: *Root:* cycloartenol, euphorbol and its hexacosanoate, taraxerone, tinyatoxin; *Bark:* euphorbol and its hexacosanate, euphorginol=taraxer-14-en-6-01, ingenol and its triacetate, taraxerone; *Latex:* a-amyrin, â-sitosterol, cycloartenol, cycloeuphordenol, 4-deoxyphorbol and its esters, euphol, euphorbinol, isoeuphorbol, palmitic acid, taraxerol, tinyatoxin, tirucallol, trimethyl ellagic acid; it may be noted that there are differences in chemical contents of latex of plant growing in differenet countries; *Stem:* campesterol, hentriacontane, hentriacontanol, kaempferol, stigmasterol, methyl ellagic acid.

Remark: The plant is worshipped as a sacred one.

FICUS RACEMOSA L. (MORACEAE)

Syn : *Ficus glomerata* Roxb.

English names: Cluster fig, Country fig, Gular fig.

Sanskrit names: Apushpaphalasambandha, Audumbaram, Brahmavriksha, Haritaksha, Hemadugdha, Shetavalkala, Udumbara, Yajnaphala.

Vernacular names: Asm : Dimoree; **Ben:** Dumur, Jajna-dumur, Jaya dumur; **Guj** : Gudar, Umar, Umbara; **Hin:** Gulav, Umar; **Kan:** Atti; **Mal:** Atti, Athimaram; **Man:** Heibong; **Mar:** Umbar(a); **Mun** : Loa daru; **Orn** : Dumbari,

Ori : Dimburi; **Sad:** Dumbair; **San:** Dumbari-hesa, Loa-dare; **Tam:** Atti, Aththi; **Tel:** Bodda, Paidi, Udumbaramu.

Trade name: Common fig.

Traditional use: *MANIPURI* : (i) *Root-extract:* in diabetes, dysentery; (ii) *Latex:* on boils; (iii) *Fruit:* in pulmonary diseases; *SANTAL* : (i) *Bark-juice:* on boils, in adenitis axillaris, epidydimitis, hydrocele, orchitis; (ii)*Latex:* on adenitis, muscular pain, pimps, scabies; (iii) *Juice of pith:* in menorrahgia, spermatorrhoea; (iv) *Warts on leaves:* in small pOX; (v) *Leaf gall (decoction)* : for washing septic wounds; *BHOXA* : *Latex:* in piles; *ETHNIC COMMUNITIES OF NORTHERN INDIA:* (i) *Latex:* in piles, pulmonary diseases; (ii) *Bark* and *Fruit* (together) : in urinary complaints; (iii) *Fruit:* as carminative; *GARHWALI:* (i) *Root:* in dysentery; (ii) *Bark:* as astringent; *ETHNIC COMMUNITIES OF MOUNT ABU* (Rajasthan): *Leaf:* in pneumonia; *ETHNIC COMMUNITIES OF CHANDRAPURA* (Maharashtra) : *Leaf:* in bronchitis; *ETHNIC COMMUNITIES OF KHEDTALUKA (Maharashtra)* : (i) Barkand *Fruit (together)* : in leprosy, urinary complaints; (ii) *Fruit:* in diabetes; *ETHNIC COMMUNITIES OF CHHINDWARA* (Madhya Pradesh) : (i) *Latex:* in diarrhoea; (ii) *Fruit:* as carminative; *ETHNIC COMMUNITIES OF BANDA* (Madhya Pradesh) : *Latex:* in dysentery, skin cracks in heels and lips.

RIGVEDA : cures piles, internal wounds, removes impurities from blood, worms from alimentary canal; *YAJURVEDA* : bark kills worms; *ATHARVAVEDA:* useful in skin diseases, including leprosy, sinus, oedema, impurities of blood and in piles; *MADANADINIGHANTU* : useful in antifertility, pimples and wounds; *BHAVAPRAKASHA* : useful in treatment of pimples and wounds; *DHANVANTARINIGHANTU* : removes worms, cures thrombophlebitis, syncope, burning sensation and unusual thirst; *KAIYADEVANIGHANTU* : astringent, sweet and heavy, cures pimples and wounds, diseases caused by deranged phlegm and deranged bile; fruits are tasteful, invigorating, astringent, cooling, cardiac tonic, useful in urinary diseases, bile disorders, menstrual disorders..

AYURVEDA: Latex: external application useful in cuts, insect bites, boils, bruises, swellings, while internal application is beneficial in haemoptysis, bleeding piles and menstrual problems.

SIDDHA : (i) *Bark:* used to prepare the drug *atti pattai,* (ii) *Latex:* for *atti pal,* and (Hi) *Leaf:* an ingredient of *atti ilai.*

Modern use: *Stem-bark* (50% *EtOH extract)* : anti-inflammatory, anti protozoal, hypoglycaemic; *Leaf-powder:* useful in bilious affections; *Leaf-gall:* beneficial in small pox.

Phytography : Spreading laticiferous tree, 9. 0-12. 2 m tall, bark reddish grey, smooth; leaves alternate, stipules ovate-Ianceolate, pubescent, 1. 25-2. 5

cm long, petioles 2. 5-5. 0 cm long, lamina simple membranous, ovate to obovate-oblong or lanceolate, 10-18 cm long, dark green, glabrous or softly pubescent above while lower surface pubescent or glabrous; fruits borne in clusters on the main trunk and leafless short branches, subglobose or pyriform, 2. 5-5. 0 cm in diameter, red when ripe.

Phenology: *Flowering:* Spring; *Fruiting:* Rainy season.

Distribution: Throughout India; Pakistan, Bangladesh, Sri Lanka.

Ecology and cultivation: Tropical plant; grows on the banks of streams, sides of ravines, on rocky slopes, up to 1500 m; wild.

Chemical contents: *Bark:* ceryl behenati gluanol-OAc, lupeol and its á-OAc, â-amyrin, â-sitosterol; *Leaf:* â-amyrin, â-sitosterol, gluanol-OAc; *Fruit:* lupeol-OAc, gluanol-OAc, glucose, hentriacontane, â-sitosterol, a sterol, ester of taraxasterol, tiglic acid.

Remarks: Some ethnic communities of Rajasthan use leaves as a galactogogue for cattle. Rural folks of Bengal, Bihar and Orissa use bark in treatment of domestic animals. Unripe fruits are eaten as a vegetable by most of the Indians, while ripe fruits are consumed by Bhoxas, Garhwalis, tribes of North-East India, hill people of Maharashtra, tribes of eastern Rajasthan, Kerala and Madhya Pradesh (Bastar).

Tribes of Chhindwara (Madhya Pradesh) use young stem as toothbrush.

This tree is considered as a constituent of the sacred *panchavata* and as *kalpataru* by the Hindus. They keep a piece of stem of this plant, as a part of rite, in the labour room and also use the wood as *samidh* (sacrificial wood) in all *yajnas.* The wood is also used by the Hindus to make effigy if the corpse is lost or not available.

GMELINA ARBOREA ROXB. (VERBENACEAE)

Syn : *Premna arborea* Roth

English names: Cashmeri tree, Coomb teak, Malay bush beech, White teak.

Sanskrit names: Ashveta, Bahdraparni, Gambhari, Gandhari, Kakodumbari, Kassmari, Katphala, Nandivriksha, Sharubhadra, Shriparni, Subhadra, Vataha, Vidarini.

Vernacular names: Asm : Gomari; **Ben:** Gamar, Gamari, Gambar; **Guj** : Shewan; **Hin:** Gamari, Gambhari, Jugani chukur, Khambheri; **Kan** : Kashmirimara, Kumbalamara, Shivani; **Lcd:** Kashmar daru; **Mal:** Kambil, Kumil, Kumilu, Kumpil; **Mar:** Shewan; **Mun** : Kasambar daru, Kasmar daru; **Orn** : Gambhair; **Ori** : Bhodroparni, Gambari; **Pun:** Gumhar; **Sad:** Gambhair; **San:** Kashmar daru; **Tam:** Gumudu-taku, Kattanam, Kumadi, Kumala maram, Perumkumbil, Umithekku; **Tel:** Gumar-tek, Gummadi.

Trade names: Gamar, Gamari, Gumhar.

Traditional use: *MIKIR: Root:* as blood purifier, *Leaf:* as carminative; *BIRHORE : Leaf:* in headache; *SANTAL* : in anasarca, asthma, bronchitis, cholera, colic pain, diarrhoea, dropsy, dyspepsia, epilepsy, fever, phthisis, rheumatism, small pox, sore, spleen complaints, syphilis, throat swelling, urticaria, as antidote to snake bite and some other poisons; *MUNDA : Bark:* to cure wounds; *SORA* (Orissa) : *Root:* in catarrh of bladder; *Decoction of root:* as tonic; *Bark:* in stomach disorder; *ETHNIC COMMUNITIES OF ARAKU VALLEY* (Andhra Pradesh) : *Root:* in malarial fever; *ETHNIC COMMUNITIES OF GODAVARI* (Andhra Pradesh) : *Bark-paste:* on bone fracture, *Leaf:* in cough, gonorrhoea; *ETHNIC COMMUNITIES OF DEHRA DUN* (Uttar Pradesh) : *Leaf-paste:* on wounds.

ATHARVAVEDA : blood purifier; *CHARAKA SAMHITA* : useful in vomiting, dropsy and in burning sensation of the body; *SUSHRUTA SAMHITA* : energiser like grape, can be used as substitute of sweet date palm; *BHAVAPRAKASHA* : it is bitter, appetiser, brain tonic, energiser, digestive, subdues *vata* and *kapha,* removes dropsy, alleviates thirst, useful in colic pain, burning sensation of body, fever, urinary complaints, wastage; *RAJANIGHANTU* : it is pungent, bitter, heavy *(guru),* thermogenic, removes oedema, phlegm, *tridosha,* burning sensation, fever, thirst, poisons; *DHANVANTARINIGHANTU* : bitter, thermogenic, removes bleeding tendency, *tridosha,* fatigue, burning sensation of body, fever, thirst; *KAIYAOEVANIGHANTU* : it is sweet, bitter, thermogenic, heavy, appetiser, digestive, brain tonic, removes dropsy, giddiness, colic pain, toxins, burning sensation of body, fever, alleviates thirst; *flowers* sweet, cooling, bitter, astringent, beneficial for the diseases caused by *pitta* and *kapha; fruits* unctuous, heavy, cooling, astringent, brain tonic, cardiotonic, removes giddiness, acidity, urinary troubles, burning sensation of body, wounds, wastage and troubles caused by *vata; RAJAVALLABHAM:* fruits seizing, bitter, sweet, heavy, cooling, good for hair, brain, removes burning sensation of body and diseases caused by *pitta; roots* are too hot; *NIGHANTU RATNAKARAM:* it is pungent, bitter, hot, astringent, heavy, sweet, appetiser, digestive, brain tonic, cardiotonic, removes thirst, colic pain, oedema, phlegm, toxins, burning sensation of body, fever, impurities of blood, piles, giddiness; *fruits* aphrodisiac, heavy, increases semen, cooling, unctuous, increases intelligence, removes urinary troubles, impurities of blood, thirst, burning sensation of body, good for urticaria, consumption, wounds, leucorrhoea.

AYURVEDA : *Root:* acrid, bitter, anthelmintic, galactogogue, laxative, stomachic, tonic, useful in burning sensation, dyspepsia, fever, haemorrhoids, hallucination, hyperdisia and stomachalgia; *Bark:* bitter, tonic, stomachic, useful in dyspepsia, fever; *Leaf-paste:* useful in cephalalgia, *Leaf-extract:* good wash for foul ulcer; *Flower:* acrid, astringent, bitter, refrigerant, sweet, useful in skin diseases including leprosy; *Fruits:* acrid, alterant, aphrodisiac, astringent, bitter, diuretic, refrigerant, sour, sweet, tonic, trichogenous, useful in anaemia, blood dysentery, constipation, leprosy, leucorrhoea, malnutrition of child and embryo, strangury and wounds.

Modern use: 50% *EtOH extract of bark* (and also of stem) : antiviral, hypoglycaemic. Phytography : Unarmed deciduous tree, 15-20 m in height; stem-bark whitish grey, lenticellate, young branches covered with fine white soft hairs; leaves. opposite, simple, petioles ±7. 5 cm long, lamina broadly ovate, usually 22. 5 by 15. 0 cm, more or less acuminate, glabrous above but stellately hairy beneath; panicles terminal, often 30 cm long, many-flowered; flowers bucciniform, brownish yellow, ±3. 7 cm long, tomentose at least when young; drupes ±1. 8 cm 1000g, fleshy, ovoid, orange-yellow when ripe; seeds hard, oblong.

Phenology: *Flowering:* January-April; *Fruiting:* May-June. Distribution: Throughout India; Bangladesh (Chittagong), Sri Lanka. Ecology and cultivation: Grows in moist deciduous forests; wild.

Chemical contents: *Root:* ceryl alcohol, gmelofuran, gmelinol, hentriacontanol-I, n-octacosanol, â-sitosterol, sesquiterpene; *Stem:* arboreok, bromoisoarboreol, cluytyl ferulate, gmelanone, gmelinol, gummidiol, lignans, lignan hemiacetal, n-hentriacontanol-I, n-octacosanol, â-sitosterol; *Leaf:* apigenin, hentriacontanol, luteoHn, quercetin, quercetogenin, â-sitosterol.

Remarks: Ethnic communities of India use the plant in the treatment of rinderpest of cattle. In Sri Lanka, it is used in skeletal fracture. It is one of the best and most reliable timber-yielding trees of India. The plant is a fast grower.

GLORIOSA SUPERBA L. (LILIACEAE)

Syn : *Methonica superba* Lamk., *Gloriosa simplex* Don.

English names: Malabar glory lily, Glory lily.

Sanskrit names: Agninukhi, Agnisikha, Ailni, Garbhaghatini, Kalikari, Lanyli, Vishalya.

Vernacular names: Asm : Utatchandal; **Ben:** Bishalanguli, Ulatchandal; **Guj** : Dudhiovachnay, Varhvareli; **Hin** : Kalihari, Kaliari, Kulhari, Languli; **Kan** : Agnisikha, Akkatangaballi, Karadikanninagadde, Kolikuttuma, Sivasaktiballi, **Mal:** Kantal, Medoni, Mattamara, Mettonsi, Mentonni; **Mar:** Bachnag, Indai, Kariannag, Khadyanag, Nagharia, Nag karia; **Mun** : Bulung chukuru; **Orn** : Jhagrahi; **Ori** : Agnisikha, Garbhhoghhatono panjanyulia, Meherlaphulo, Panchaangula; **Pun:** Kariari, Mulim; **Sad:** Jhagar; **San:** Siricsamano; **Tam:** Akkinichilam, Kalappaikkilanku, Kalaippaikkishangu,

Kannuvalikkodi, Nabhikkodi, **Tel:** Adabhinabhi, Agnisikha, Gangeri, Kalappagadda.

Traditional use: *ETHNIC COMMUNITIES OF NORTH-EAST INDIA: Root:* in gout, stomachache and as tonic; *MUNDA AND ORAON: Tuber:* for antifertility purpose; *SANTAL* : (i) *Tuberous root:* for abortion purpose, in intermittent fevers, wounds; (ii) *Plant:* in spleen complaints, syphilis, tumours; (ii) *Leaf:* in asthma; *ETHNIC COMMUNITIES OF BIHAR: Root:* in cholera, to facilitate childbirth; *ETHNIC COMMUNITIES OF ORISSA: Tuber* : as abortifacient; *TRIBES OF VARANASI* : *Root:* in gout; *TRIBES OF PITHORAGARH: Tuber:* in gonorrhoea, leprosy, piles; *ETHNIC COMMUNITIES OF DEHRA DUN AND SIWALIK: Root:* as anthelmintic; *ETHNIC COMMUNITIES OF GARHWAL* : *Tuberous root:* for abortion;

CHARAKA SAMHITA : useful in itching, skin diseases including wounds and ailments caused by vitiated *kapha* (phlegm) and *vata* (wind); *SUSHRUTA SAMHITA:* can be administered to a delivered mother along with spirituous drink to give relieve to her postnatal complaints, *roots* are poisonous; *RAJANIGHANTU:* it is pungent, thermogenic, eliminates deranged *kapha* (phlegm) and *vata* (wind), terminates pregnancy; *DHANVANTARI NIGHANTU:* in addition to the above, it is also useful in dropsy, labour pain, wounds, and as a purgative; *MADANADI NIGHANTU* : it is bitter, pungent, thermogenic, abortifacient, removes abdominal pain, expels the placenta, cures phlegm, skin diseases; *BHAVAPRAKASHA* : it is apperient, alkaline, astringent, pungent, bitter, highly potent, light, abortifacient, helps storing up energy, excites *pitta* (bile), it cures dropsy, piles, wounds, acute spasmodic pain, and removes worms; *CHAKRADATTA* : *Root-paste:* if smeared over' the palms and feet of a pregnant woman, delivery of child becomes easier.

AYURVEDA : (i) *roots* are abortifacient, acrid, alexiteric, anthelmintic, antipyretic, bitter, depurative, digestive, emetic, expectorant, gastrointestinal irritant, highly poisonous, purgative, rejuvenating, stomachic, thermogenic, tonic, beneficial in vitiated conditions of *kapha* (phlegm) and *vata* (wind), debility, dyspepsia, flatulence, haemorrhoids, helminthiasis, inflammations, in promoting labour pain and expulsion of the placenta; (ii) *root-paste* is effective against paralysis, rheumatism, snake bite, insect bites; (iii) *leaf-juice* effective against lice.

Modern use: *Root* (aq. extract) : ecbolic in humans and other animals; *Plant* (50% *EtOH extract)* : spasmolytic, Central Nervous System depressant; *Leaf-juice:* piscicide. **Phytography** : Herbaceous tendril climber; rootstock tuberous, naked; stem 3-6 m long, sparingly branched; leaves sessile or nearly so, opposite or 3-nately whorled, tip tendrillar; flowers axillary, solitary, nearly 10 cm, at first greenish, becoming yellow and finally scarlet or red; capsules nearly 5 cm long.

Phenology: *Flowering:* October; *Fruiting:* throughout the year.

Distribution: Throughout tropical India ascending up to 2000 m on the hills; Indo-China, Malaysia.

Ecology and cultivation: Plains from the coast on thickets; wild.

Chemical contents: *Root:* colchicine, b-sitosterol and its glucoside, band t-lumicolchicine, 2-0H-6-MeO benzoic acid; *Young leaf:* cholidonic acid; *Flower:* luterlin and its glucosides, N-formyl-de-Ac-colchicine, lumicolchicine; *Seed:* colchicine.

Remarks: It is getting less attention in India, though extensive researches are on abroad.

GYMNEMA SYLVESTRE R. BR. EX SCHULT (ASCLEPIADACEAE)

Syn : *Periploca sylvestris* Willd., *Gymnema melicida* Edgew.

English names: Vine, Periploca of the the woods.

Sanskrit names: Ajaballi, Ajagandini, Ajashringi, Bahalchakshu, Chakshurabahala, Grihadruma, Karnika, Kshinavartta, Madhunasini, Medhasingi, Meshashringi, Meshavishanika, Netaushadhi, Putrashringi, Sarpadanshtrika, Tiktadughdha, Vishani.

Vernacular names: Ben: Meshashringi; **Guj** : Dhuleti, Mardashing; **Hin** : Gurmar, Gumar, Merashinghi; **Kan** : Karhasige, Sannagera-shehumbr; **Mal:** Cakkarakkolli, Madhunashini; **Mar:** Kavali, Kalikardor, Vakundi; **Tam:** Adigam, Cheorukurinja, Kannuminayamkodi, Pasaani, Sakkaraikkolli, Shirukurinja, Sirukurumkay; **Tel:** Podapatra.

Trade names: Gurmar, Merasingi.

Traditional use: *KOL* : *Leaf:* in gastric troubles; *ETHNIC COMMUNITIES OF RAJASTHAN* and *DHASAN VALLEY: Leaf:* in diabetes; *ETHNIC COMMUNITIES OF KANDALA* (Maharashtra) : *Leaf:* in urinary complaints; *GOND: Leaf:* in diabetes, stomachache; *ETHNIC COMMUNITIES OF MADHYA PRADESH: Leaf:* in cornea opacity and other eye diseases; *ETHNIC COMMUNITIES OF GODAVARI DISTRICT* (Andhra Pradesh) : *Leaf:* in diabetes, glycosuria; *IRULAR* : *Leaf:* in diabetes; *CHARAKA SAMHITA:* removes bad odour from breast milk, aperitive; *SUSHRUTA SAMHITA* : *plant* useful as purgative, in eye troubles; *leaf extract* and also the same of *flower* beneficial for eyes; *bark* useful in the diseases caused by vitiated *kapha* (phlegm); *BAGBHAT* : *rootbark* useful in piles; *BHAVAPRAKASHA:* it is bitter, appetiser, gastric stimulant, removes cough, alleviates breathing troubles, useful in curing phlegm, eyetroubles, wounds; *RAJA NIGHANTU* : appetiser, removes phlegm, piles, colic pain, cures dropsy, useful in eye troubles, cardiotonic, beneficial in respiratory diseases, wounds, detoxicant; *fruits* are bitter, sialagogue, thermogenic, cures the diseases caused by vitiated *kapha* (phlegm) or *vata* (wind); *NIGHANTU RATNAKARAM* : removes cough, vitiated wind, detoxicant, appetiser, useful in eye troubles. *AYURVEDA* : acrid, alexipharmic, anodyne, anthelmintic, antipyretic, astringent, bitter, cardiotonic, digestive, diuretic, emetic, expectorant, laxative, stimulant, stomachic, uterine tonic; useful in amennorrhoea, asthma, bronchitis, cardiopathy, conjunctivitis, constipation, cough, dyspepsia, haemorroids, hepatosplenomegaly, inflammations, intermittant fever, jaundice and leucoderma; *root* emetic and removes phlegm; external application is useful in insectbite;

SIDDHA : an ingredient of 'Cirukuricinver'; *UNANI* : an ingredient of 'Gurmarbuti'.

The fresh leaves, when chewed, paralyse the sense of sweet for sometime; for this reason it is called *gur-mar,* thereby meaning sugar-killer and impression has become prevalent in some parts of the country that it is useful in *diabetes mellitus.* Chewing fresh leaves also paralyse the taste of bitter for a while.

Modern use: *Aerial parts* (50% *EtOH extract)* : spasmolytic, hypyoglycaemic, *in vitro* antiviral against influenza A2 virus.

Phytography : Stout, woody, large climber; young branches slender and pubescent; leaves opposite, simple, petioles 0. 6-1. 2 cm, stout or slender, lamina 2. 5-6. 25 cm in length, elliptic or ovate, thinly coriaceous, upper surface rarely pubescent; cymes subglobose, ± 1. 25 cm in diameter; flowers yellow, ±0. 2 cm in diameter; follicles slender, ±5-7. 5 by 0. 8 cm; seeds pale brown, flat, ±1. 25 cm long.

Phenology: *Flowering:* August-March; *Fruiting:* Winter.

Distribution: Mainly in Deccan peninsula, also found in Madhya Pradesh, Maharashtra, Rajasthan; Sri Lanka.

Ecology and Cultivation: Grows in the plains from the coast, in scrub jungles and in thickets; wild.

Chemical contents: *Leaf:* conduritol A, gymnestrogenin, gymnamine, hentriacontane, nonacosane, penta-OH-triterpene.

Remark: In Sri Lanka, plant used in bone fractures.

GINKGO BILOBA L. (GINKGOACEAE)

English name: Maiden hair tree.

Vernacular name: Hin : Balkuwari.

Trade name: Ginkgo.

Traditional use: *Seeds:* expectorant and sedative.

Modern use: *Tanakan* (active principle of plant extract) : effective in induced cerebral ischemia in rats; *Tebonin* (a preparation containing leaf extract) : used in cardiovascular disorders, increased cerebral blood circulation, Parkinson's disease; *Nut* (extract) : antibacterial against *Mycobacterium smegmatis.*

Recently *Ginkgo* is rapidly gaining recognition as a brain tonic that increases memory and boosts oxygen level in brain. It regulates neurotransmitters, increases blood flow and metabolism. It reduces migraine and vertigo. It may be useful in mental disorders, including Alzheimer's disease. Recently a pill containing extracts from *Ginkgo* has been launched for eliminating excess fat (cellulite) in women.

Phytography : Tree with pyramidal form, reaching a height of 30 m; leaves petiolar, lamina fan-shaped, bilobed; dioecious; mature seeds orange-coloured and are about the size of an apricot.

Phenology: *Flowering* and *Fruiting:* Summer.

Distribution: Darjeeling (West Bengal).

Ecology and cultivation: Native of China, cultivated in Indian gardens, particularly on hills.

Chemical contents: *Root-bark:* Ginkgolides A, B, C & M; *Plant:* bilobalide, bilobanone sesquiterpene; *Leaf:* flavonols, biflavonoids, diterpenes, sesquiterpene bilobalide A, â-sitosterol, ginkgolides A, B & C, shikimic acid, sequoyitol, 1, 5-MeO-bilobetin; *Fruit:* anacardic acids, ginnol, bilobols, cardanols.

Remarks: Chinese consume *Ginkgo* seeds. Endosperm of roasted seed is edible and kernel is highly nutritious. It is believed that regular consumption of *Ginkgo* preparation staves of ravages of age and checks senility. *Ginkgo* is a contemporary of dinosaurs of the Jurassic period. Because of its primitive characters, it is known as living fossil. It is a native of Chekiang in East China. It is grown by the Buddhist monasteries of China and Japan as a sacred tree. The plant was introduced into Europe in early 18th Century and later in America. Only a few trees occur in India. Perhaps it does not exist in the wild today. Because of its nutritional and medicinal properties, it is receiving increased attention. Commercial cultivation of this species should be endeavoured in India. If appropriate measures for conservation of this important medicinal species are not taken, it is destined to be extinct in the near future.

GARCINIA XANTHOCHYMUS HOOK. F. EX T. ANDERS (CLUSIACEAE)

Syn : *Xanthochymus tinctorius* DC., *Garcinia tinctoria* Dunn.

English name: Egg tree.

Sanskrit names: Tamala, Tapinjha.

Vernacular names: Ben: Tamal, Chalta; **Hin** : Dampel, Tamal, Tumul; **Guj** : Kasamala, Ota; **Kan:**Deva-garige; **Mal:** Anavaya; **Man:** Heilbung; **Mar:** Jharambi, Dampel, Ota; **Nep** : Chunyel; **Ori** : Cheoro, Sitambu;

Tam: Kulavi, Malaippachai, Mukki, Tamalam; **Tel:** Sitakamraku, Evarumidi, Tamalamu.

Trade name: Tamala.

Traditional use: *Fruit:* antiscorbutic, cooling, digestive, emollient, demulcent and cholagogue. *Sherbet* made from dried fruit is used in billiousness.

AYURVEOA : *Young branch:* paste as ointment on boils; *Bark:* astringent; *Leaf:* decoction useful in diarrhoea; *Young leaves* (roasted in a special method) : used in dysentery; *Seed:* butter made from seeds useful in pulmonary affections, dysentery, goitre.

Modern use: *Xanthochymol* : antibacterial against *Streptococcus faecallis* and *Klebsiella pneumoniae.*

Phytography : Evergreen tree, trunk straight; branches arising in tiers, drooping, angular; leaves opposite, coriaceous, bright green, shining, 22. 5-45. 0 cm by 5-10 cm; flowers polygamous, male flowers from axils of fallen leaves, fascicled with 4-8 flowers, white, thick, rough, hermaphrodites like male flowers, ovary ovoid, usually 5:chambered; fruits subglobose, pointed, dark yellow; seeds 1-4, oblong, yields a large quantity of gamboge.

Phenology: *Flowering:* Spring; *Fruiting:* Summer.

Distribution: Native to India and Myanmar; distributed widely in the lower hill forests of eastern Himalaya, Meghalaya, Sikkim, West Bengal, Maharashtra, Gujarat, Tamil Nadu, Kerala, Andhra Pradesh, the Andamans; Bangladesh, Myanmar.

Ecology and cultivation: Tropical forest; wild.

Chemical contents: *Fruit:* xanthochymol, isoxanthochymol, maclurin, euxanthone, 1, 5-dihydroxy-and 1, 3, 5-trihydroxy-xanthones, methoxyxanthones, cambogin, volkensiflavone, morello-flavone, biflavones.

Remark: In South India, fruits of this species are used in lieu of tamarind.

HOLARRHENA PUBESCENCE (BUCH. -HAM.) WALL EX DC. (APOCYNACEAE)

Syn : *Holarrhena antidysenterica* (L.) Wall., *Echites pubescens* Buch. -Ham.

English names: Bitter oleander, Conessi bark, Dysentery rosebay, Easter tree, Ivory tree, Tellichery bark.

Sanskrit names: Girimallika, Indrayava, Kalinga(ka), Kalingyava, Katuka, Katuja, Mahagandha, Mallikapushpa, Panduradruama, Pravrishya, Sangrahi, Shakrapadapa, Vatsika, Vrikshaka, Yavaphala.

Vernacular names: Asm : Dhurkhuri, Ducikhuri; Ben: Kurchi, Katuraj, Kuteswar, Indrajava; Guj : Dhowda, Kuda, Kari; Hin : Kurchi, Karchi, Karra; Kan : Beppale coodsaloo, Korchie; Lep : Fajeerip; Mal: Kodagapala; Mar: Kura, Kala-kura, Kear, Kewar, Kodago, Kuda, Dola-kuda, Pandhrakura; 'Mun :

Ludu-ba, Toa-ba; Nep : Khuria; Ori : Kherwa, Pita, Korwa, Patru kurwa; Orn : Koraia; Pun: Kawar, Kura, Kear, Kewar; Sad: Koraia; San: Hat; Tam: Kuda-sappalai, Veppalei, Kodagapalei, Indrabam; Tel: Kodisepala, Palakodsa, Pala, Kodaga.

Trade name: Kurchi.

Traditional use: *MANIPURI* : Bark (boiled extract) : in diarrhoea, dysentery; GARO : Bark and Leaf: in dysentery; *ETHNIC COMMUNITIES AROUND GUAHATI:* Seed: as anthelmintic; *BODO* (of Assam) : Bark: in diarrhoea, dysentery, piles; Flower: as appetiser and in intestinal worms; Seed.. in leprosy; *ASUR* (of Bihar) : Bark: in snake bite; Seed: diarrhoea, fever, intestinal worms; *MUNDA* : Root and Leaf: in diarrhoea, bleeding from nose, haemorrhage after childbirth; *SANTAL* : Root: in bite of dog or jackal, blood and mucous in bowel excretion, diarrhoea, dysentery, hematuria, spermatorrhoea, spleen complaints; Bark.. in bronchitis, chameleon's bite, cholera, cold, colic, fever, menorrhagia; Fruit: in anaemia, colic, constip5ltion, diarrhoea, dry cough, epilepsy, gravel, postnatal complaints, stomachache; *TRIBAL SOCIETIES OF HAZARIBAGH AND RANCHI* : Bark: in gastric disorder, to revive taste in tongue; *ETHNIC COMMUNITIES OF ORISSA*: Latex: in eczema and other skin diseases; *ETHNIC COMMUNITIES OF ABUJH-MARH* (Madhya Pradesh) : Bark: in menstrual complaints; *TRIBAL COMMUNITIES OF SAGAR* (Madhya Pradesh) : Seed: in dysentery; *THARU* (of Uttar Pradesh) : Bark: in fever; Bark and Seed (together) : in dysentery; KOL (of Uttar Pradesh) : Seed: in digestive complaints; *ETHNIC COMMUNITIES OF DEHRA DUN AND SIWALIK*: Seed: in diarrhoea, dysentery, fever; *ETHNIC COMMUNITIES OF EAST RAJASTHAN*: Bark and Seed (together) : in dysentery; *ETHNIC COMMUNITIES OF MOUNT ABU*: Bark: as antidote to snake bite; *DANG*: (of Gujarat) : Bark: in diarrhoea; *VASAVA* (of Gujarat) : Root: in fever; Root and Bark (together) : in gout; *ETHNIC COMMUNITIES OF SAURASHTRA*: Bark: in bronchitis; *ETHNIC COMMUNITIES OF DAHANU FOREST DIVISION* (Maharashtra) : Bark and Leaf (together) : in dysentery; Latex: as antidote to snake bite, Seed: in asthma, colic.

ATHARVAVEDA : increases semen, tightens the slackened muscles; *CHARAKA SAMHITA* : Bark (paste) : good for skin diseases, leprosy, ringworm, piles, fistula, adenitis; Fruit: in vomiting, beneficial in disorders caused by vitiated phlegm and bile, as galactagogue; Seed: in piles; *SUSHRUTA SAMHITA*: Flower: beneficial in deranged phlegm and bile, and a good remedy for leprosy; *CHAKRADATTA*: Bark: in diarrhoea; *BHAVAPRAKASHA:* pungent, drying, refrigerant, excitant, cures piles, diarrhoea, phlegm, bile, leprosy, alleviates thirst; *RAJANIGHANTU* : pungent, bitter, thermogenic, astringent, cures diarrhoea, vitiated bile, skin diseases and piles; *DHANVANTARINIGHANTU*: pungent, bitter, astringent, drying, cooling, cures skin diseases, gastroenteritis, vitiated bile; *MADANANIGHANTU* : excitant, digestive, astringent, beneficial in bleeding tendency, worms, skin diseases; *SALIGRAMNIGHANTU* : appetising, beneficial in vitiated phlegm, cures diarrhoea, skin diseases, worms; *KAIYADEVANIGHANTU* : astringent, cooling, drying, excitant, pungent, beneficial in vitiated phlegm, bile, skin diseases, diarrhoea, piles; Flower: refrigerant, bitter, astringent, excitant.

AYURVEDA: Bark and Seed: acrid, anthelmintic, antiperiodic, aphrodisiac, astringent, bitter, carminative, expectorant, febrifuge, stimulating, beneficial in asthma, bronchitis! blood dysentery, diarrhoea, dropsy, dysentery, fever, haemorrhages, haemorrhoides, hepatopathy, malaria, piles, rheumatism, skin diseases, urinary troubles, verminosis, vomiting; Leaf: useful in boils, bronchitis, dysentery and wounds.

SIDDHA: Root and Bark: used as constituents for the preparation of Kutacap patai.

UNANI : in the preparation of Sufuf Habis and Majnum Bawasir.

Modern use: Bark (50% EtOH extract) : hypotensive; Bark-powder: in abdominal and glandular tumours; Fruit (50% EtOH extract) : anticancer, anti protozoa, hypoglycaemic, astringent, febrifuge, useful in diarrhoea, intestinal worms, and to regulate menstruation.

Phytography : Deciduous tree or large shrub; leaves sessile or subsessile, broadly ovate to elliptic-oblong, abruptly acuminate, often unequal, rounded or obtuse at base, lateral nerves 10-15 pairs, arching near the margin; flowers white, bracts small, follicles 20-42 by 0. 8-1. 2 cm; seeds up to 1 cm long, linear-oblong, coma about twice as long as seeds, seeds brown.

Phenology: Flowering and Fruiting: May-January.

Distribution: Major parts of India up to 1500 m in the Himalaya; Bangladesh, also in Africa-mostly in drier regions.

Ecology and cultivation: Common in village surroundings; sometimes in private gardens. Chemical contents: Root-bark: holacetine; Stem-bark: L-quebrachitol, dihydroisoconessimine, kurcholessine, 3-a-aminoconan-5-ene, 7-a-OH-conessine, holonamine; Leaf: aminoglycosteroids, aminode-oxyglycosteroids, kurchiphylline, kurchiphyllamine, kurchaline, holadysine, holadysamine, holantosines A, B, C & D, holarosine A, B, E & F.

Remarks: Tribals of East Rajasthan give root to cattle in a disease in which tongue ejects out and gets swollen. Tribals of Maharashtra eat flower and seed as vegetables. Ethnic communities of Ratan Mahal Hills use latex to curdle milk. Santal women use flowers to decorate their hairdos. Tribals of Madhya Pradesh use wood to make combs and many household articles.

5

Traditional Systems of Medicinal Plants

SOME IMPORTANT MEDICINAL PLANTS USED IN TRADITIONAL SYSTEM OF TREATMENT

In India the popularity of the herbal medicine formulated by various Indian scholars went unabated up to 1940s that is till the beginning of modern allopathic system of medicine. It is worthwhile to mention briefly the medicinal properties of some common plants used in ayurvedic system of medicine.

1. TULASI: *(Occimum sanctum)* Tulasi is not only most popular holy plant in Indian household but also proved to be a 'Wonder Drug' against all sorts of cough and cold problems. Tulasi symbolises sanctity and purity
2. YASTIMADHU: *(Glycirrhiza glabra)* Yastimadhu or Licorice is a very popular name in Ayurvedic system of medicine. It is used as restorative, urinary tract sedative and against cough and cold.
3. VASAK: *(Justicia-Adhatoda Vasika)* It is a household remedy for cough and cold and its leaf extract is used in anti-cold preparation.
4. NEEM: *(Azadiracta indica)* Like Tulasi Neem is also a holy plant and its fruit kernels, leaves and barks used in traditional Ayurvedic medicine as potent antimicrobial agents. The chewing of neem twig is very popular practice in India to fight tooth decay and gum troubles.
5. GUGUL:*(Commiphora mukul)* & RASNA *(Vanda roxbergii)* Gugul is a resinous substance exuded from Gugul plant which has potent anti-rheumatic and anti-cholesterol activity. Rasna extract is very effective against Gout and all kinds of Rheumatism. Both Gugul and Rasna are widely use in all anti-rheumatic preparations and found to be very effective.

6. TRIFALA: (Amla, Haritaki, Bahera) This trio are super megastar in Ayurvedic system of medicine and are used as all disease fighter and prophylactic against a host of diseases like constipation, dyspepsia, liver troubles etc.
7. ASHWAGANDHA: *(Withania somnifera)* Ashwagandha is a single super star in the field of health restorative like *Panax ginseng* of Korea. It finds application in many Ayurvedic formulation.
8. ARJUN: *(Terminalia arjuna)* -The extract of Afjun bark is a well proven anti-hepertensive drug and well established as a Cardiac Tonic.
9. SHANKHAPUSHPI: *Evolvulus occinoides)* -Shankhapushpi is found all over the country in rainy season in open grass land or on stony wasteland. Its sharbat is beneficial in mental fatigue and memory revitalising. It has also anti-pyretic property. It has the reputation in curing mental disorder. A team of scientists of BHU proved that shankhapushpi is very good against haemotemesis and hypertension.
10. ARNI :(Sans. *Agnimantha, bot. -Clerodendrum phlomidis)* In south India its leave juice is used to treat gonorrhea and syphilis. Adivasis, particularly, Santals rub the plant over their body in dropsy.
11. BRAHMI: (*Bacopa monnieri*-Linn*)* The plant is well known for its potency to increase one's memory and said to improve intellect, used against epilepsy I insanity and other nervous disorders. The leaves are used as diuretic and aperients and contain alkaloids like brahmine and herpestine and saponin-hersaponin which showed cardiotonic action in frog.
12. PUNARNAVA: *(Boerhavia diffusa) :* Punarnava is one of the major constituents of many ayurvedic medicines. It is well known in Indian house-hold for its medicinal properties. Roots of *B. diffusa* considered to be a potent expectorant, diuretic and laxative. It is also used in asthma. Fairly good diuretic in dropsy associated with bright's disease. The drug exerts more powerful action as compared to other diuretics on certain types of ascites such as those of liver and chronic peritonitis. Active constituent of *B diffusa* is punarnavine.
13. PIPPALI: *(Piper longum)* : Fruits are used as spice and also used as preservative in pickles. Roots and fruits are used against diseases of respiratory tract. It is also used as analgesic and anti-inflammatory in muscular pain. It also posseses the properties like sedative, carminative, cologogue in obstruction of bile duct and gall bladder. In Indian house-hold powder of dried fruit is taken with honey for relief from common cold and cough.
14. GOKSHURA OR IKSHUGANDHA :*(Tribulus terrestris)* : Leaves and tender shoots are used as pot herb. Fruits are source of flour used in

times of scarcity. Leaves are rich in calcium, but poor in iron supplying cheap supplement to rice diets. Fruits are used in ayurvedic as tonic and diuretic. It is used in painful micturition and urinary calculus. It is also prescribed in bright's disease. Herb contains saponins such as diosgenin, gotogenin, chlorogenin, ruscogenin, and 25 D-spirosta-3, 5-diene.

15. NIRGUNDI:(*Vitex negundo*) : Leaves are used as tonic and vermifuge; smoked for relief from cold and catarrh and headache. Leaves and root possess tranquilizing effects and form a constituent of famous ayurvedic preparation Vishagarbha taila. Extract of leaves show anti-cancer activity against Ehrlich ascites tomour cell. Root is used as tonic, febrifuge and in rheumatism. It is also used as demulcent in dysentry and piles. Flowers are used in liver complaints, fever and diarrhoea.
16. MANDUKAPARNI: (*Centella asiatica*) : It is a diuretic and tonic. It is also use in treatment of leprosy. A glycoside-asiaticoside proven to be the active principle in treatment of leprosy has been isolated scientists.
17. SHATABARI: (*Asperagus recemosus*) : A very common name in ayurveda and widely used as tonic in ayurvedic medicines. It is also used as diuretic and galactogogue. Fresh root juice is mixed with honey and given for dyspepsia. Roots form a constituent of medicinal oils for nervous and rheumatic complaints.
18. VIDARI: (Oriya-*Bhuin Kakharu. bot. -Ipomoea mauritiana*) : Tuberous roots contain a resin similar to Jalap resin and are considered tonic, aphrodisiac, demulcent, lactagogue and cholagogue. Powdered root is given in diseases of spleen and liver, debility, fatty deposition and menorrhagia.
19. MADHUNASHINI: (*Gymnema sylvestra*) : Leaves, when chewed paralyse for few hours the sense of taste for sweet and bitter substances. In ayurveda, G. *sylvestra* is being used as anti-diabetic drug with doubtful integrity. Leave powder is cardiac stimulant and diuretic..
20. ASHOKA: (*Saraca asoka syn-*S. *indica*) : Ashoka is a well known medicine in ayurveda for treatment of uterine disorders. Due to its stimulating effect on endometrium and ovarian tissue and hence it is useful in menorrhagia due to uterine fibroids. Flower is used as uterine tonic. It is also used in biliousness, heamarrhagic dysentry.
21. MANDUPARNI OR COMMON YEW: (*Taxus baccata*) :'Leaves and various parts of the tree possess anti-cancer property. Taxus leaves and its parts are being exported from Northern states to USA and France for preparation of anti-cancer and anti-malarial drugs. Many of the ayurvedic preparation contain manduparni which is becoming rare due to its export demand..

22. GULUCHI: (*Tinospora cardifolia*) : Stem is a constituent of several ayurvedic preparations used in general debility, dyspepsia, fever and urinary diseases. Dry twigs with bark intact constitute the drug. The bitter principle present in the drug show anti-spasmodic, anti-pyretic and anti-inflammatory properties. The decoction of guluchi plant is given in gout. The drug possesses one fifth of the analgesic effect of aspirin.
23. CHITRAKA: (*Plumbago indica or zeylanica*) Root is abortifacient, vesicant, and diuretic and used in dyspepsia, piles, diarrhoea and skin diseases. The paste of root is applied in opening of abscesses. Infusion of roots used in influenza and black-water fever.
24. GHRITA KUMARI: (*Aloe barbadensis; syn* A. *vera*) : A well known medicine plant in India. Fresh juice of leaves is cathartic and refrigerant and used in liver and spleen diseases and in eye troubles. It is believed to cool the brain-therefore it is used as a hair tonic. Leaf extract inhibits the growth of mycobacterium tuberculosis. It is found to be useful in X-ray burns, dermatitis and cutaneous leishmaniasis and other skin disorders. The jelly of *Aloe vera* is being used by many Multi National companies in their sun ray protecting creams. Its jelly is now found to be a good culture medium for tissue culture. It will cut down the cost of culture medium which is being exported from foreign countries.
25. GAMBHARI: (*Gmelina arborea*) : It is found in the forests of Orissa plentily. Its wood is used for furniture making. Its root is one of the constituents of well known and well tested ayurvedic tonic called Dashamularishta.
26. MITHIPATTI (*Scoparia dulcis*) : In Bastar region it is called *Mithipatti or Ghodatulsi* Infusion of the leaves used in fever, cough and bronchitis. Its juice is used as gargle in toothache. Anti-diabetic compound, amellin, occurs in the leaves and stems of green plants. It is helpful in anaemia, albuminaria, ketonuria, retinitis associated with diabetes.
27. PASHANABHEDAKA (*Homonoia riparia*; Oriya *Jamla,* Tam. -*Kattalari)* : Root laxative, diuretic, used in piles, stone in bladder and vesicle calculi, strangury, and !Jsed in urinary discharges. Tender leaf is used as vegetables.

ACTIVE HYPOGLYCEMIC CONSTITUENTS FROM PLANTS

Many active compounds have been isolated from the plant and herb species of India. These active principles are dietary fibres, alkaloids, flavonoids, saponins, amino acids, steroids, peptides and others. These have produced potent hypoglycemic, anti-hyperglycemic and glucose suppressive activities.

The above effects achieved by either insulin release from pancreatic â-cells, inhibited glucose absorption in gut, stimulated glycogenesis in liver or increased glucose utilization by the body. These compounds also exhibited their antioxidant, hypolipidemic, anticataract activities, restored enzymatic functions, repair and regeneration of pancreatic islets and the alleviation of liver and renal damage. Some active constituents have been obtained from plants possess insulin like activity and could be provide alternate for insulin therapy. Chemical structures of few active compounds having anti-diabetic potentials from above mentioned plants are provided.

Metabolic imbalance causing diabetes mellitus is a characteristic of materialistic world. Differences in social structure, psychic stress, obesity, hormonal imbalance and heredity are optimizing the growth of pandemic. Increasing population with diabetes has a huge requirement of effective remediation.

The Indian flora has a vast variety of medicinal plants, which are used traditionally for their anti-diabetic property. However, careful assessment including sustainability of such herbs, ecological and seasonal variation in activity of phyto-constituents, metal contents of crude herbal anti-diabetic drugs, thorough toxicity study and cost effectiveness is required for their popularity.

These efforts may provide treatment for all and justify the role of novel traditional medicinal plants having anti-diabetic potentials.

BIO-INFORMATICS ON MEDICINAL PLANTS AND TRADITIONAL KNOWLEDGE

Medicinal Plants Master Database

A comprehensive master database on medicinal plants of India has been systematically built up at FRLHT over the last 8 years. Currently, this database incorporates more than 7, 500 botanical names which are linked to more than 1, 40, 500 vernacular names in 13 different languages like Tamil, Kannada, Malayalam, Hindi, Sanskrit, etc. Each such correlation can be traced back to a published reference.

This database also incorporates more than 10, 000 authentic digital images of plants duly linked to their botanical names. An important feature of this database is a fully-referenced distribution database which provides information on geographical distribution of nearly 6, 000 plant species. Through a system of assigning a unique ID number to each botanical name and linking various aspects of information, for each species, to this unique ID, data relating to several different aspects like propagation, trade, pharmacognosy etc can be quickly accessed for a specific plant entity with search being initiated with the help of a botanical or vernacular name.

This multi-faceted database forms the backbone for undertaking and promoting sustainable use and informed conservation action for native medicinal plant species and also acts as a platform for designing various research projects relating to the management of this valuable natural resource.

This database is also linked to referenced information on the plant materia-medica of traditional systems of medicine as well as to pharmacognosy and pharmacology of the plant entities.

PHARMACOGNOSY DATABASE ON INDIAN MEDICINAL PLANTS

A computerised database called Labguru has been created for storing and retrieving referenced literature on pharmacognosy and pharmacology of medicinal plants. Labguru is a stand-alone database with an easy-to-use interface, linked to the master database.

This database is a valuable literature source for researchers and industry alike. Data compilation is from published sources such as texts and on-line databases. This is an ongoing evolving activity in the laboratory at FRLHT.

Database on metals and minerals used in Indian medicines

Mineral and metal medicine is used by traditional practitioners all over India. These are potent medicinal materials which need accurate identification of materials and careful processing for their proper use.

Therefore it was decided to develop a user-friendly and easily retrievable database on mineral and metal medicine by compilation of relevant references from authentic traditional texts of Ayurveda that are difficult to procure at one place for most users. Correlating the traditional names of metals minerals to modern geological entities helps to understand the identity of the minerals used.

AYUSH Databases

FRLHT in the last 10 years has been documenting and developing traditional knowledge databases on the materia medica of Indian systems of medicine.

Medicinal plant databases have been already initiated on Ayurveda, Siddha, Unani system and Homoeopathy. The current FRLHT databases have screened a limited number of the known medical texts written across the period 1500 BC to 1900 AD and therefore much work yet remains to be done.

In the next 5 years we would also like to initiate new database work on diagnostics and other speciality areas like *panchakarma* and *rasayana*, as these fields are critical for effective application of Ayurveda and Siddha. The main goal of the databases is to serve the needs of students and teachers of Indian systems of medicine, medical practitioners, researchers, community enterprises, community health NGOs and pharmaceutical companies.

Database of plants of Susruta Samhita

The database of plants of Susruta Samhita has 9, 650 references. This data has been converted from the previous data environment to the present one to support access to various database tools. A checklist of the plant names was prepared and a report is made available in Sanskrit and English scripts.

Database on plants of Siddha medicine

The bilingual database has an extensive collection of information pertaining to a therapeutic information of plants mentioned in 5 texts of 2, 350 records, simple remedies mentioned in 6 texts of 1, 800 records, formulation data of 3, 013 records and 36, 000 records of dictionary file which has Tamil names of plants.

A separate nighantu file in Tamil script and a glossary of the technical terms are also incorporated in this database.

Database on plants of Homoeo medicine

This database could complete compilation of plants and products information of 80 plants mentioned in Homoeo medicine from 15-20 sources as text document.

Database on plants of Unani medicine

A hard copy of the Arabic and Urdu names appearing in the classical texts of Unani medicine was prepared from the FRLHT's nomenclature database. Verification on botanical names and spellings of Arabic names and Unani names were carried out.

DATABASES FOR ASSESSMENT OF LOCAL HEALTH TRADITIONS

The web-based Referral Browser basically aims to provide support for assessment of folk health traditions. This will help to promote best health-related practices in a specific area for human, plant and animal health care. The browser will procure references from Ayurveda, Siddha, Unani and modern pharmacology for a resource used in folk health practice and is subjected to evaluation/assessment.

SPECIALISED REPORTS & CHECKLISTS

FRLHT has come out with state wise checklists and specialised reports on medicinal plants in conservation sites. While specialised reports have been prepared and published on the medicinal plants of Karnataka, Kerala and Tamil Nadu, checklists have been prepared for Andhra Pradesh, Maharashtra, Madhya Pradesh, Arunachal Pradesh, Himachal Pradesh, Meghalaya and Uttranchal. The specialised reports list the species recorded in the state and the species found in the MPCAs, their habit and the system of medicine in which they are used. Specialised reports also has the distribution and the forest type maps of the respective state, the botanical profile of the state and the MPCA and the habit wise analysis of the medicinal plants.

INFORMATION PRODUCTS

CDs on Medicinal plants of southern India

Three CDs on medicinal plants of Karnataka, Kerala and Tamil Nadu have been designed for the use of researchers working in the field of conservation. The CDs incorporate data on checklist of medicinal plants in each of these States. It also provides information on threat status of the species, synonyms, different systems of medicine they are used in and forest type where the plants occur. There are around 900 images. Information is also available on primary health care uses for 128 species and propagation techniques for 200 species. More than 65, 000 regional names have been included, in different languages like Sanskrit, Hindi, Marathi, Telugu, Kannada, Malayalam and Tamil, along with maps to show the occurrence of individual species in various forest types. The search of a species can be done either from botanical or regional name. It can filter the species depending on the forest type, threat status, system of medicine and by the language.

Clinically Important plants of Ayurveda (CIPA)

Clinically Important Plants of Ayurveda is now available as a CD-ROM, which contains detailed information of 3500 pharmaceutical preparations for 200 indications. It has plant pictures, botanical and regional names, Sanskrit synonyms and its complete reference, plant properties and English meaning of all technical Sanskrit terms. This would be useful for pharmaceutical industries, Ayurveda practitioners and researchers.

Plants of Caraka Samhita

This bilingual database incorporates 12, 873 plant references from Caraka Samhita which are grouped into 620 species. This was carried out based on a guideline prepared for grouping plant names as anonyms, synonyms and variant names. In the database, each plant reference is provided with its English translation and all the technical terms are supported with a dictionary of its English meaning. Classification of medicinal plants, 1, 700 formulation information, plant picture, various botanical correlations and its identity status, habit and trade information of selected species, commentator's opinion of plant identity, etc. are the important features of this database.

A multimedia CD was designed with necessary visual effects highlighting the importance of Caraka Samhita. A brochure on this CD is also available to support dissemination activities.

Database on plants of Ayurveda for BAMS course

All classical information pertaining to detailed and non-detailed list of plants mentioned in the BAMS (Bachelor of Ayurvedic Medicine and Surgery) syllabus were compiled from 20 classical texts. There are 370 plants in the syllabus which are incorporated in the database. Botanical names, regional names, classical references like Sanskrit slokas, interpretation of the slokas into English, and usage of these plants as single drugs are incorporated into this database.

Modern botanical information such as morphology, distribution, propagation methods and pharmacognosy information inclusive of its plant biochemistry and pharmacology are provided. This database is aimed to provide all required information for graduates and postgraduate students of Ayurveda.

Database on Ayurveda formularies

The database of the Ayurveda formularies incorporated in the Ver. 1 of CIPA (Clinically important plants of Ayurveda) CD. The second version of the CIPA will have 4, 000 more Ayurvedic formulation compiled from 7 classical texts covering about 150 plants.

TRIALS FOR ANTI-DIABETIC POTENTIALS OF MEDICINAL PLANTS

Recently the plants and herbs are being used as decoctions or in other extracted forms for their blood sugar lowering potential. There are some useful reviews on Indian medicinal plants having blood sugar lowering potentials. Many useful herbs introduced in pharmacological and clinical trials have confirmed their blood sugar lowering effect, repair of â-cells of islets of Langerhans. Details of some potent Indian herbs, their recently reported pharmacological and clinical hypoglycemic efficacy, active chemical constituents, their mechanism of action and available toxicity status are described chronologically as follows:

AEGLE MARMELOS LINN. COOREA (FAMILY: RUTACEAE)

Hindi name: Bel; Common name: Holy Fruit Tree

The trees grow throughout deciduous forest of India and ripen fruits are commonly use for delicacy. *Aegle marmelos* is widely used in Indian Ayurvedic medicine for the treatment of diabetes mellitus. Hypoglycemic effect of root bark decoction (1ml/100mg) has been observed in normal fasted rats. Leaf extract produced anti-hyperglycemic activity in alloxan diabetic rats along with decreased cholesterol and blood urea. In diabetic rats leaf extract exhibited insulin like activity. Aqueous leaf extract has been shown to improve the functional state of pancreatic cells in streptozotocin induced diabetic rats. Aqueous leaf extract (250 & 500mg/kg, orally) produced hypoglycemic effect and increased plasma insulin level of STZ-diabetic rats. LD_{50} (lethal dose) observed greater than 10. 0g/kg at oral administration to rats. Anti-hyperglycemic activity caused by leaf extract (250mg/kg, orally) in glucose fed hyperglycemic rats (Sachdewa *et al.*, 2001). Aqueous fruit extract (250mg/kg, twice daily for one month) produces anti-hyperglycemic effect along with decreasing glycosylated haemoglobin level in STZ induced diabetic albino wistar rats. Hypoglycemic and antioxidant activity of leaves have been observed in diabetic male albino rats. Fruit extract (125 and 250mg/kg, orally twice daily for 30 days) produced anti-diabetic, anti-hyperlipidaemic and antioxidant activity in STZ diabetic rats along with partial repair of damaged pancreatic islets (Kamalakkanan *et al.*, 2005). Treatment of severely (fasting blood glucose level >250 mg/ml) diabetic rats for 14 days with aqueous extract (250mg/kg, orally) of *Aegle marmelos* seeds reduced the fasting blood glucose by 60. 84% and urine sugar by 75% than their pretreatment levels.

ALLIUM CEPA LINN. (FAMILY: LILIACEAE)

Hindi name: Pyaj; Common name: Onion

The plant is cultivated throughout India. Onion bulb and leaves are the important part of diet. Ether soluble fraction of onion (0. 25mg/kg, orally) has been observed to lower blood sugar level in normal rabbits and exhibited potent antioxidant activity (Auguati, 1973). In a clinical study treatment of diabetic patients by juice of *Allium cepa* bulb, controlled the blood sugar level. Dipropyl disulphide oxide and onion oil produced significant hypoglycemic effect. Significant blood sugar lowering produced by petroleum ether extract (2g/kg) from onion bulb in glucose, induced hyper-glycemic rabbits. A sulphur containing amino acid, S-methyl cystein sulphoxide (at a dose of 200mg/kg for 45 days) from onion showed potent hypoglycemic activity in alloxan induced diabetic rats. S-allyl cystein sulphoxide from onion significantly reduced blood glucose level of alloxan induced diabetic rats. Prolonged administration of freeze dried onion powder (3%) with a diet produced anti-hyperglycemic, hypolipidemic and antioxidant activity in STZ-diabetic rats. Onion callus cultures showed greater hypoglycemic potential over natural onion bulb. Prolonged administration of a diet containing onion produced hypoglycemic and antioxidant effect in diabetic rats. *Allium cepa* juice (0. 4g/ 100g b. w. for 4 weeks) exhibited anti-hyperglycemic and antioxidant effect in alloxan induced diabetic rats, it also repaired hepatic and renal damage caused by alloxan.

ALLIUM SATIVUM LINN. (FAMILY: LILIACEAE)

Hindi name: Lahsun; Common name: Garlic

The plant is cultivated all over India. It is an important part of dietary ingredients. Allicin (0. 25mg/kg, orally) from garlic exhibited pronounce hypoglycemia in mild diabetic rabbits. In alloxan induced diabetic rabbits ethanol, ethyl acetate and petroleum ether extract (0. 25mg/kg, orally) produced antihyperglycemic activity. Treatment of alloxan diabetic rats with the antioxidant s-allyl cysteine sulfoxide isolated from garlic ameliorates the diabetic condition almost to the same extent as did glibenclamide and insulin. It also significantly stimulates *in vitro* insulin secretion from â-cells isolated from pancreas of normal rats. Extract (500mg/kg/day) of *Allium sativum* bulb proved to be effective for treatment of l-thyroxine (l-T4) induced hyperglycemia in rats. Alloxan induced diabetic rats fed a diet containing *Allium sativum* (12. 5%) for 15 days were able to reduce blood glucose as compare to control group. Oral administration of a laboratory diet containing 0. 05% of ajoene (derived from garlic) for 8 weeks has been observed to produce anti-diabetic effect in genetically diabetic KK-A(y) mice. The levels of plasma glucose significantly suppressed about 73. 8%. Two garlic compounds garlic oil (100mg/ kg body weight) and diallyl trisulfide (40mg/kg body weight) given every other day for 3 weeks to STZ-diabetic rats significantly raised the basal insulin concentration and increased the insulin sensitivity. Herbal extract of garlic (20mg 100 g-1 body weight, orally, daily for 5 weeks) produced hypoglycemia, probably by interfering with food intake of both normal and STZ-diabetic rats. S-allyl cysteine, a key component of aged garlic, found potent antioxidant and inhibited AGEP (accumulation of advanced glycation end products) formation. Bis (allixinato) oxovanadium (IV) from garlic found to be the most potent anti-diabetic agent in type 1 diabetic mice on both intraperitoneal injections and oral administrations (Adachi *et al.,* 2006).

ALOE VERA (LINN.) BURM. F. (FAMILY: LILIACEAE)

Hindi and Common name: Aloe

The herbs are cultivated throughout India for its variety of medicinal properties. Dry sap of plant produced prominent anti-hyperglycemic response in type 2 diabetic patients (½ teaspoonful, orally for 4–14 weeks), and in alloxan induced diabetic Swiss albino mice (500mg/kg, twice daily for 5 days). In a clinical study, it was reported that oral administration of aloe might be a useful adjuvant for lowering of blood glucose in diabetic patients. *Aloe vera* leaf pulp extract showed hypoglycemic activity on type 1 and type 2 diabetic rats, the effect being enhanced in type 2 diabetes as compared with glibenclamide. Plant extract (200 and 300mg/kg, orally) produced hypoglycemic activity along with controlled carbohydrate metabolizing enzymes in normal fasted, oral glucose fed and STZ-diabetic rats. Oral administration of ethanolic extract (300mg/kg b. w.) to STZ-diabetic rats for 21 days resulted in a prominent reduction of fasting blood glucose along with improved plasma insulin level of diabetic rats. Administration of the five phytosterols from *Aloe vera* namely, lophenol, 24-methyl-lophenol, 24-ethyl-lophenol, cycloartanol and 24-methylene-cycloartanol to severe type 2 diabetic mice for 28 days decreased the fasting blood glucose levels 64%, 28%, 47%, 51%, and 55% respectively. Oral administration of *Aloe vera* gel extract (300mg/kg b. w. per day for 21 days) to STZ-diabetic rats resulted in a significant reduction of fasting blood glucose and improved the plasma insulin level.

ANDROGRAPHIS PANICULATA (BURM. F.) NEES (FAMILY: ACANTHACEAE)

Hindi name: Kalmegha; Common name: King of Bitter

This is an annual herb that grows throughout India. Plant extract effectively produced hypoglycemic and anti hyperglycemic activity in normal rats. Different doses (0. 1, 0. 2, and 0. 4g/kg b. w.) of plant extract effectively reduced the fasting serum glucose level of STZ-diabetic rats. Antihyperglycemic and antioxidant activity of plant extract (400mg/kg b. w, twice a day for 14 days), has also been reported in diabetic rats. The andrographolide from plant increases the glucose utilization and lowers plasma glucose in diabetic rats lacking insulin. Significant reduction in blood glucose level (52. 90%) observed when hyperglycemic rats treated with 50mg/kg body weight aqueous extract of *Andrographis paniculata*. This effect enhanced when freeze-dried material used at a dose of 6. 25 mg/kg body weight, it reduced 61. 81% blood glucose level. The anti-diabetic potentials of plant restored the impaired estrous cycle in alloxan-induced diabetic rats.

ANNONA SQUAMOSA LINN. (ANNONACEAE)

Hindi name: Sharifa; Common name: Sugar apple tree

The plants grow throughout India and commonly use by tribal communities of Northern India for the treatment of diabetes. Aqueous leaf extract produces hypoglycemic activity in streptozotocin-nicotinamide induced diabetic rats. Ethanolic leaf-extract (350mg/kg b. w., orally 10-day) administration to STZ-diabetic rats has been shown to lower fasting blood glucose level to (73. 3%), and treatment of severely diabetic rabbits with leaf-extract (350mg/kg, for 15 days) reduced fasting blood glucose by 52. 7% and urine sugar by 75%. *Annona squamosa* fruit pulp extract (2. 5 and 5. 0g/kg b. w.) has been observed to improve the glucose tolerance of alloxan diabetic rats. Further more, fruit pulp (5g/kg b. w.) brought down urine sugar, urine protein and glycol-hemoglobin in diabetic rabbits. Oral administration of aqueous leaf-extract to diabetic rats for 30 days significantly reduced the levels of blood glucose and increased the activity of plasma insulin and antioxidant enzymes.

AZADIRACHTA INDICA A. JUSS. (FAMILY: MELIACEAE)

Hindi name: Neem; Common name: Indian lilac tree

This is an evergreen tree grows throughout India. Aqueous extract is known to produce antihyperglycemic and hypoglycemic activity in diabetic dogs. Fresh leaves decoction induced antihyperglycemic activity and increased the peripheral glucose utilization in normal rats. Leaf extract of *Azadirachta indica* has been reported to produce the hypoglycemic activity in normal rats without altered serum cortisol level (Chattopadhyay *et al.*, 1999). Crude ethanol extract (250mg/kg, for 2 weeks) potentially lowered the blood sugar level of alloxan diabetic rats.

Leaf extract has been observed to produce anti-hyperglycemic activity in streptozotocin diabetic rats without altered serum cortisol level. Petroleum ether extract of seed kernel (2gm/kg b. w.) & seed husk (0. 9gm/kg b. w.) restricted oxidative stress in heart and erythrocytes caused by streptozotocin in diabetic rats. Dianex, a polyherbal formulation consists of the aqueous extract of *Azadirachta indica* has been well tolerated in laboratory animals at higher doses (up to 10 g/kg in mice, acute toxicity; up to 2. 5 g/kg in rats, sub-acute toxicity studies for 30 days) without any toxic manifestation. Beta-sitosterol, a steroid obtained from *Azadirachta indica,* may be responsible for its hypoglycemic property. In a clinical study of type 2 diabetes powdered part, aqueous extract and alcoholic extract of *Azadirachta indica* at high dose for 14 days exhibited hypoglycemic activity.

CINNAMOMUM TAMALA (HAMM.) NEES. & EBERM. (FAMILY: LAURACEAE)

Hindi name: Tejpat; Common name: Bayberry

The plant is cultivated in different parts of India and use as spice. Aqueous leaf extract induced potential blood sugar lowering effect in 18 hours fasted and glucose induced hyperglycemic rabbits at a dose of 500mg/kg. Oral administration of powdered leaves (20gm for 15 days) exhibited hypoglycemic effect in patients of type 2 diabetes mellitus along with insulin released from pancreatic â-cells. In a clinical study, leave powder produced hypoglycemic response in type 2 diabetic patients. Ethanolic extract (210mg/kg) of leaves induced potential hypoglycemic effect in 18 hours fasted albino rats. Alcoholic extract of leaves produced hypoglycemic activity in alloxan induced diabetic rats when administered orally for two weeks at a dose of 250mg/kg.

COCCINIA GRANDIS (LINN.) VOIGT (FAMILY: CUCURBITACEAE)

Syn. *Coccina indica* (White & Arn); Hindi name: Kunderi; Common name: Ivy Guard

The plants are wild creepers grow in many parts of India. Blood sugar lowering effect has been observed in patients treated with homogenized freeze dried leaves. Ethanol extract (250mg/kg) of whole plant produced hypoglycemic activity in fasted, glucose fed and diabetic albino rats. Hypoglycemic effect of alcoholic extract (250mg/kg, orally) of *Coccinia indica* was observed in fasted and glucose fed hyperglycemic male albino rats. Alcoholic leaf extract produced hypoglycemic effect in normal fed and 48 hours fasted rats, response mediated by suppression of gluconeogenic enzyme glucose-6-phosphatase. Pectin (200mg/100gm/day) isolated from fruits, exhibited blood sugar lowering effect and an increase in the glycogen content of liver in normal rats. Ethanol (60%) leaf extract (200mg/kg, orally) lowered the blood sugar level of diabetic rats due to suppressed glucose synthesis, through depression of glucose-6-phosphatase, fructose-1-6-biphosphatase and enhanced glucose oxidation by shunt pathway through activation of glucose-6-phosphate dehydrogenase. Leaf extract was produced hypoglycemic, and insulin secretogouge activity in diabetic patients. Dried extract (500mg/kg, p. o. for 6 weeks), of plant exhibited anti-hyperglycemic activity in diabetic patients. Extract mimic insulin like activity and improved the functional status of enzymes in glycolytic pathway and lypolytic pathway. Potent antioxidant and hypolipidemic activity exhibited by ethanolic leaf extract administered at a dose of 200mg/kg for 45 days to streptozotocin induced diabetic rats.

FICUS BENGALENSIS LINN. (FAMILY: MORACEAE)

Hindi name: Bargad; Common name: Indian Banyan Tree

Plants grow throughout India and in the Indian tradition it is considered as a holy tree. In a chronic toxicity test extract (25 & 250mg/kg), produced reversible hepatic damage while the acute LD_{50} (lethal dose) found to be 9. 47g/kg body weight when given intraperitoneally. Leucocyanidin (3-O-â-D-galactosylcellobioside) a dimethoxy derivative isolated from bark, lowered blood sugar level and increased serum insulin in normal and moderate diabetic rats. It also inhibits the degradation processes of insulin. Alcoholic extract of stem bark at a dose of 25, 50 & 75mg/day/100g, b. w. lowered the blood sugar level 47 to 70%, and also restored the normal levels of serum urea, cholesterol and total protein of alloxan diabetic albino rats.

Glucoside of leucopelargonidin isolated from bark has been reported to induce hypoglycemic, hypolipidemic and serum insulin raising effect in moderately diabetic rats. 3-O-alfa-L-rhamnoside (250mg/kg, single dose study & 100mg/kg/day, long term study), a dimethoxy derivative isolated from bark, lowered blood sugar in fasted and glucose induced hyperglycemic rats, along with enhanced insulin secretion from â-cells.

Leucodelphinidine derivative isolated from bark exhibited hypoglycemic activity in normal and alloxan diabetic rats. 3-O-á-L-rhamnoside isolated from the bark has been showed its median effective dose (ED_{50}) as 100mg/kg with 12% hypoglycemic action in normal rats. Hypoglycemic and hypercholesterolemic effect of aqueous bark extract was observed in alloxan induced mild and severe diabetic rabbits. Lethal dose (LD_{50}) of this was found to be 1gm/kg, when administered orally for 3 months in rats. Leucopelrgonin (100mg/kg/day for one month) isolated from bark lowered the fasting blood sugar (34%) and glycosylated haemoglobin (28%) of alloxan diabetic dogs.

GYMNEMA SYLVESTRE (WILLD) R. BR. (FAMILY: ASCELPIADACEAE)

Hindi name: Gudmar; Common name: Periploca of the wood

Plants are grown in tropical regions of India and used as household remedy for diabetes. Oral administration of a water soluble fraction G-54 isolated from *Gymnema sylvestre* administered to 27 type 2 diabetic patients reduced their insulin requirement, lowered the fasting blood sugar and glycosylated haemoglobin content. Two water soluble fractions (GS-3 and GS-4) obtained from leaves were found to double the pancreatic islets and â-cell numbers in diabetic rats. Alcoholic leaf extract (500mg/kg, orally) lowered maximum blood sugar in fasted, glucose fed and diabetic rats along with insulin released from pancreatic â-cells. In rats the insulin secretion from islets of Langerhans and several pancreatic â-cell lines induced by alcoholic extract in absence of other stimulus.

Gymnemic acid IV, isolated from leaves produced potent hypoglycemic effect in STZ-diabetic mice. Leaf extract has been observed to produce anti-hyperglycemic and hypoglycemic effects of in corticosteroid-induced diabetes mellitus, without altered serum cortisol concentration. A polyherbal formulation containing aqueous extracts of *Gymnema sylvestre* produced prominent hypoglycemic activity in normal and diabetic rats at a dose of 100–500mg/kg/day, orally for acute, 6 hours and for long-term, 6 weeks studies. Gymnemic acid IV isolated from the leaves has been observed to produce hypoglycemic, anti-hyperglycemic, glucose uptake inhibitory and gut glycosidase inhibitory effects.

MOMORDICA CHARANTIA LINN. (FAMILY: CUCURBITACEAE)

Hindi name: Karela; Common name: Bitter gourd

The plant is an annual climber grown mostly in tropical India and commonly use as vegetable. Charantin (50mg/kg, orally) isolated from *Momordica charantia* has been resembled insulin lower blood sugar level (maximum 42% at 4th hour) of rabbits. In a clinical study of type 1 and type 2 diabetic patients the polypeptide-p isolated from fruit, seeds and tissue exhibited hypoglycemic activity without any side effect.

The subcutaneous injection of (0. 5unit/kg) lowered the blood sugar in gerbils and langurs. Charantin obtained from *Momordica charantia* induced hypoglycemic effect and also stimulated the insulin release and blocked the formation of glucose in blood stream. Hypoglycemic effect and delayed cataract development was reported in alloxan diabetic rats treated with fruit extract (4g/kg/Day orally for 2 months). Ethanolic extract (200mg/kg) of *Momordica charantia* was produced hypoglycemic activity in normal and streptozotocin diabetic rats; this was occurred possibly due to inhibiting glucose-6-phosphatase and fructose-1, 6-biphosphatase in liver, and stimulating hepatic glucose-6-phosphate dehydrogenase activities. Oleanolic acid and momordin from plant, produced antihyperglycemic effect by inhibiting glucose transport in intestine of rat. Fruit aqueous extract (200mg/kg, orally for 6 weeks), and exercise potentially lowered blood sugar of type 2 diabetic and hyperinsulinemic (insulin resistance) rats. Seed aqueous extract produced prominent reduction in blood glucose, glycosylated hemoglobin, lactate dehydrogenase, glucose-6-phosphatase, fructose-1, 6-bisphosphatase and glycogen phosphorylase along with increased hemoglobin, glycogen content and hexokinase, glycogen synthase activity. Anti-diabetic properties of plant such as charantin, vicine and polypeptide-p have the potential to be a part of dietary supplement for patients of diabetes. From *Momordica charantia* the major compounds, 5b, 19-epoxy-3b, 25dihydroxycucurbita-6, 23(E) -diene(4) and 3b-7b, 25dihydroxycucurbita-5, 23(E) -dien-19-al(5) administered at a dose of 400mg/kg produced hypoglycemic effect in ddY mice strain.

OCIMUM SANCTUM LINN. (FAMILY: LAMIACEAE)

Hindi name: Tulasi; Common name: Holy Basil

It is a tropical annual herb grown all over India and use for household remediation. Oral administration of alcoholic extract of leaves of *Ocimum sanctum* lowered blood sugar level in normal; glucose fed hyperglycemic and STZ-diabetic rats, along with increased insulin release. *Ocimum sanctum* leaf powder was produced potent hypoglycemic and hypolipidemic effect in normal and diabetic rats. Alcoholic extract of leaves significantly lowered the blood glucose in normal and alloxan diabetic rats. Administration of plant extract 200mg/kg in STZ-diabetic rats for 30 days led to decreased in plasma glucose level by 26. 4%. Plant extract lowered blood glucose level along with inhibited cortisol level. From leaf extract the aqueous butanol and ethylacetate fractions stimulated insulin secretion from perfuse rat pancreas, isolated rat islets and a clonal rat â-cell line in a concentration-dependent manner.

PTEROCARPUS MARSUPIUM ROXB. (FAMILY: FABACEAE)

Hindi name: Vijayasar; Common name: Indian Malabar

Plants grow throughout India and are use as hypoglycemic plant in folklore medicine. Aqueous bark extract lowered blood sugar and improved glucose tolerance of diabetics with no side effects observed. From alcoholic extract of bark the ethyl acetate soluble fraction caused blood sugar lowering and repaired the alloxan induced pancreatic â-cells damage in albino rats. From plant the (-) -epicatechin (30mg/kg, i. p.) produced anti-hyperglycemic effect in alloxan induced diabetic rats. The (-) epicatechin, from bark increased the cAMP content of the pancreatic islets associated with increased insulin release, conversion of proinsulin to insulin and cathepsin B activity in rats. Marsupin and pterostilbene, two phenolic constituents of plant potentially lowered blood glucose at same level as compared to metformin in STZ-diabetic rats. Aqueous extract (1g/kg, orally) of bark has been observed to produce anti-cataract activity in alloxan diabetic rats. Plant extract was prevented the hyper-triglyceridaemia and hyper-insulinaemia (insulin resistance) in type 2 diabetic patients. Aqueous extract (250mg/kg, orally) of dried wood has been reported to produce hypoglycemic effect in acute and sub-acute study.

SWERTIA CHIRAYITA (ROXB. EX FLAM) KARST. (FAMILY: GENTIANACEAE)

Hindi name: Kirayat Chirata; Common name: Bitter Stick

The herbs grow abundantly in Himalayan regions of India and are used for treatment of various ailments by the tribes. 95% ethanol extract (250mg/kg) of plant potentially lowered the blood sugar level in fasted, glucose fed and tolbutamide pretreated animals. Hexane fraction (250mg/kg, b. w. orally for 28 days) of plant, lowered blood sugar of albino rats with increased glycogen content of liver and insulin released from pancreatic â-cells. Swerchirin (50mg/kg, orally) isolated from hexane fraction of plant exerted potent hypoglycemic activity in normal and STZ-diabetic albino rats. A xanthone isolated from the hexane fraction of *Swertia chirayita* identified as swerchirin (1, 8-dihydroxy-3, 5-dimethoxyxanthone) exhibited blood sugar lowering effect in fasted, fed, glucose fed hyperglycemic and tolbutamide pretreated albino rats. Effective dose (ED_{50}) of *Swertia chirayita* has been reported to be 23. 1mg/kg/oral, lower maximum 40% blood sugar level of male albino rats of body weight 140–165g. Swerchirin (50mg/kg, b. w. orally) isolated from crude extract lowered maximum 60% blood glucose at 7 hour post-treatment, along with depleted aldehyde-fuchsin stained b-granules and immunostained insulin of islets of Langerhans. Swerchirin isolated from plant was found to be superior blood sugar lowering agent over tolbutamide. Alcoholic extract (250mg/kg, once daily for two weeks) exhibited hypoglycemic effect in alloxan induced diabetic rats.

SYZYGIUM CUMINI LINN. (FAMILY: MYRTACEAE)

Syn. *Eugenia jambolana* (Linn.); Hindi name: Jamun; Common name: Black Berry

Plants grow in different parts of India. The ripe fruits are used as part of dietary component. Oral administration of fruit pulp induced hypoglycemic activity in normal and STZ-diabetic rats along with insulin released from â-cells. Seed powder provided good symptomatic relief to 30 patients of diabetes (type 2) and regulated blood sugar level. Increased activity of hexokinase and decreased activity of glucose-6-phosphate in liver produced blood sugar lowering effect at oral administration of aqueous seed extract (2. 5g/kg, b. w. for one month) to alloxan diabetic rats.

Aqueous seed extract (2. 5 & 5g/kg, b. w. for 6 weeks) has been observed to produce hypoglycemic and antioxidant activity, and increase in haemoglobin content in rats. Alcoholic seed extract injection (20mg, intraperitoneally) reduced the blood sugar level to 37. 17% at 3 hour and 46. 68% at 6 hour of administration in alloxan diabetic mice along with enhanced insulin secretion. Decreased plasma glucose concentrations in STZ-induced diabetic mice was observed at oral administration of fruit extract (200mg/kg, for 50 days).

Blood sugar lowering, hypolipidemic activity, increased serum insulin, increased glycogen content of liver and muscles and a fall in glycosylated haemoglobin level produced by ethanolic extract (100mg/kg b. w. orally) of seed.

Ethanolic seed kernels extract (100gm/kg b. w.) has been observed to improve glucose tolerance, and produce hypoglycemic and hypolipidemic effect in STZ-diabetic rats. *Syzygium cumini* was produced prominent fall of blood sugar in mice. Aqueous and ethanolic extracts of the fruit-pulp has been reported to produce antihyperglycemic effect in alloxan diabetic rats, and 24. 4% raise in plasma insulin level in mild diabetic and 26. 3% in severely diabetic rabbits.

TRIGONELLA FOENUM-GRAECUM LINN. (FAMILY: FABACEAE)

Hindi name: Methi; Common name: Fenugreek

Plants are commonly cultivated throughout India. The leaves are used as vegetable and seeds as spice. Major alkaloid trigonellin from fenugreek seeds produced hypoglycemic activity. Ethanol extract (0. 8g/kg, i. p.) of leaves has been observed to reduce blood glucose concentration in alloxan induced diabetic rats. Lethal doses (LD_{50}) of aqueous leaf extract were 1. 9g/kg at intra-peritoneal and 10g/kg at oral administration. 4-Hydroxyisoleucine, an insulinotropic compound isolated from seeds increased the insulin release in glucose fed hyperglycemic rats and humans.

Seeds powder treatment normalized the enhanced lipid peroxidation and reduced the susceptibility to oxidative stress associated with depletion of antioxidants in liver of rats. Maximum 46. 64% decrease in blood sugar level of diabetic rats was observed at oral administration of seed extract (1g/kg, for one month).

From fenugreek seeds, the soluble dietary fibre (SDF) fraction at (0. 5g/kg, orally administered twice daily, for 28 days) inhibited platelets aggregation in type 2 diabetic rats and produced beneficial effect in dyslipidemia.

Restored activity of glutamate dehydrogenase, NAD linked isocitrate dehydrogenase and D-b-hydroxybutyrate dehydrogenase reported at oral administration of seed powder (5%, for 3 weeks) in alloxan diabetic rats. It also repaired the liver and kidney damage caused by alloxan. 4-hydroxyisoleucine:5, an amino acid, isolated from seeds, produced anti-hyperglycemic effect and decreased the 33% plasma triglyceride, 22% total cholesterol (22%) and 14% free fatty acids.

RECENT RESEARCH ON MEDICINAL PLANTS & REVIVAL OF HERBAL MEDICINE

Being convinced that modern allopathic medicines, though potent, are not safe and also being convinced that these drugs are not sustainable in the context of its incompatibility in the natural system the gamut of modern allopathic drugs is being reviewed differently in recent past. The revival of herbal medicines and its productive blending with modern medical science have been given serious thoughts. The recent findings on the properties of medicinal plants are very amazing. Here we may mention a few of such findings.

A: ON HUMAN

1. SADABAHAR :. The most common Indian plant Sadabahar whose botanical name is *Catharanthus rosea syn-Vinca rosea* found to contain an important cytotoxic alkaloids vincrystin in smaller quantity and vinblastin in larger quantity. Vincrystin found to be clinically effective against leukemia and vinblastin against Hodkin diseases. The credit goes to USA and Canadian scientist who initiated resJ3arch in 1950s on isolation of alkaloids from common Rosy Periwinckle or *Catharanthus rosea or vinca rosea.* After the discovery of vincrystin the survival rate of children suffering from leukemia has jumped over to about 80 %. The clinical effectiveness of vincrystin in leukemia among children created a huge demand for Vinca rosea in USA.
2. ASHWAGANDHA: A team of Doctor from Kasturba Medical College, Manipal have reported that an alcoholic root extract of Ashwagandha has shown anti-tumour activity. They have also reported that Ashwagandha Injection can also augment the effect of radiation on tumor regression and delayed its growth.
3. RAKTA CHITRAKA: The same team led by Prof. P. Umadevi also reported that the extract of Rakta Chitraka (*Plumbago Indica)* a well known herbs in traditional Indian medicine found to have effective anti-tumor property and augmenting the effect of radiation given concurrently in arresting the growth of Tumour. Rakta Chitraka is being prescribed for cancer treatment in Siddha system.
4. MUSTARD : Mustard a popular condiment and oil-seed in India may have potential anti-cancer property according to a preliminary study at the National Institute of Nutrition, Hyderabad. Such anti-cancer property may be attributed to chemical compound phenyl-iso thiocyanate present in mustard seed.
5. NEEM: Extensive researches in India well as abroad on Neem *(Azadiracta*

Indica) has opened new vistas in Herbal medicines due to its versatile-properties.

Neem extract has shown activity against Rodent-Malaria caused by *Plasmodium berghei* prevalent in West Africa according to Scientist of University of Nizeria and African Bio-Science Net Work. Researches are being continued to investigate the activities of Neem and other plants against deadly parasite, *Plasmodium falcifarum,* found in African countries.

Indian researches on versatile applications of Neem are very promising. It is an established fact the chewing of Neem twig fights mouth Bacteria/ protozoa causing tooth decay, Gingivitis and Pyorrhea. India is the first country to manufacture Neem-based tooth paste and soap.

It has been found by the scientist of Defense Institute of Physiology and Science (DIPAS) and National Institute of Immunology (NII), New Delhi that Neem oil acts as an effective spermicidal contraceptive without any hazardous side effects. The contraceptive formulation called Nm-76 prepared from Neem oil extract which is undergoing trials and expected to be a safe and effective vaginal-spermicide. NIL scientist have clinically tried two Neem based products-PRANEEM OIL & PRANEEM POLYHERBAL CREAM which are effective as vaginal contraceptive and vaginal anti-microbial.

A team of Indo-American scientist from NII, New Delhi and Harvard Medical School, USA have shown that a sugar like extract from Neem bark can stop infectivity of AIDS-VIRUS in human blood cells, cultured in laboratories. No doubt, this findings may bring a new hope in the treatment of AIDS.

A group of researchers have shown Neem leaves extract acts as a sedative and anxiolytic in low dose of 10 to 200 mg/kg of body wt. in experimental rate.

Scientists of Malaria Research Institute New Delhi have reported that Neem oil is an excellent and low cost mosquito repellent. 5% Neem oil mixed with kerosene burnt in lamp. repels mosquitoes effectively without causing any harm to human body, unlike mosquito repellent mats and coils. A cream developed from Neem oil when applied to human body nullify the bites of sand fly that spreads Kalazar prevalent in Bihar.

B: ON PLANTS

Recently it has become a serious concern that the chemical pesticide leave high percentage of residual poison in the edible agro-horticultural product leading to serious health hazards. This is one of the bad effects of so called green revolution. Now it is high time that we should seriously think about alternative pesticides and. fungicide which are safe both to human and environment.

It is a matter of pleasure that such alternative pesticides are heading their way by the dedicated efforts of scientist and in near future these will come in a big way and may totally replace the hazardous chemical pesticide. These may be called as bio-pesticide which are of two types: 1) Microbe-based and 2) Plant Extract-based. As we are presently concern about the medicinal plant, we may cite a few examples where plant extracts are processed as pesticides.

1. Extract of marigold leaves (Electra of Ecomax Agrotech) is effective against soil nematodes and it is used as soil spray.
2. Aqueous extract of neem seed powder when sprayed on plants can effectively control a number of plant insects and fungal infections.
3. REPLIN-a spray insecticide formulation enriched with neem extract prepared by ITC agro-Industry, Hyderabad successfully tested in the field and found to be effective against steam borer and leaf folders.

C: ON ANIMAL

Even the veterinary surgeon depends upon plant for the treatment of the animal. Scientist from Calcutta have discovered anti-filarial activity in a drug isolated from the plant *Acacia auriculoformis.* The drug contains two active compounds acaciaside A and acaciaside B. These two saponins at a concentration of 4 mg. per ml. killed 97 percent of micro-filaria-the slender pre-larval forms of the filarial nematode in 100 minutes. The compound could also kill all the adults in 35 minutes. This report is published by the scientists ion the Indian journal of experimental biology.

NATIONAL RESEARCH INSTITUTES ON MEDICINAL PLANTS

Following R & D labs. and institution are engaged specifically on identification, isolation of chemicals and improving agro technique for cultivation of medicinal plants.

1. Central Institute for Medicinal-Lucknow & Aromatic Plants (CIMAP).
2. National Botanical Research Institute. -Lucknow
3. Regional Research Laboratory-Jorhat, Tiruvantpuram, Bhubaneswar, Jammu.
4. Central Drug Research Inst. -Lucknow
5. Council for Scientific and Industrial Research (CSIR) -New Delhi

MEDICINAL PLANTS AS A SOURCE OF RAW MATERIALS FOR ALLOPATHIC MEDICINE

Besides the direct applications of extract, powder, seed powder etc. of medicinal plants on the diseases, as mentioned in traditional system of medicines, many medicinal plants are used in pharmaceutical or drug industries to extract intermediary raw materials in manufacturing of various allopathic medicines.

1. There are sorrye plants which contain 4 to 8 % of diosgenins, the steroidal saponins and examples being *Diascorea floribunda, Dioscorea deltoidea* the common yam or khamb-alu in Oriya. Diosgenins when subjected to appropriate chemical reactions converted to cortisone a steroidal hormones for therapeutic purposes..
2. Reserpine an alkaloid extracted from Rouwlfia serpentina root (Sarpagandha) is used for manufacturing anti-hypertensive and sedative drugs.

TO CONSERVE AND CULTIVATE MEDICINAL PLANT-A GLOBAL NEED

It is now a need to preserve the medicinal plant which are in this spasm of extinction and to cultivate medicinal plants on commercial basis due to the following reasons.

1. It is being observed that many useful 11ledicinal plants have become either endangered or becoming extinct particularly in the tropical eco-system of developing countries. It is apprehended that the modern allopathic system of medicine will suffer a serious set back if certain medicinal plant species go totally extinct. Therefore, it is high time that our policy makers should seriously think about the preservation of such species in the form of herbarium and Gene Bank.
2. Increased demand for medicinal plants like Sadabahar, Rouwlfia, Occimum sanctum, Neem, Ashwagandha, Panax ginseng etc. warrants a development of improved agro-techniques for large scale commercial cultivation in tropical countries. It is interesting to know that there is a substantial demand from Ayurvedic. Allopathic and Homeopathic medicine manufacturers for medicinal plants. The estimated demand of various medicinal plants from leading Ayurvedic medicine manufacturer alone in India like Charak, Zandu. Dabur, Baidyanath etc. amounts to about Rs. 1000 crores per year. The export demand in India for Vinca rosea for preparation of vincrystin in USA is about RS. 5 million.
3. The justification for commercial cultivation for medicinal plants may also be attributed to rampant deforestation.

CULTIVATION OF MEDICINAL PLANTS- A NEW ENTREPRENEURIAL OPPORTUNITY IN RURAL AREAS

Commercial cultivation of most demanded medicinal plant will lead to sustainable employment generation in the rural and tribal areas of India *vis-a-vis* enormous ur. 1employment problem and secondly it will boost up our forex earning through export ultimately both leading to over all economic development. Therefore, it may be concluded without any doubt and ambiguity that cultivation of medicinal plants offers an opportunity for entrepreneurial venture in a big way, particularly for S & T entrepreneurs.

AN OVERVIEW OF INDIAN NOVEL TRADITIONAL MEDICINAL PLANTS WITH ANTI-DIABETIC POTENTIALS

Diabetes mellitus is the most severe metabolic pandemic of the 21st century, affecting essential biochemical activities in almost every cell in the body and increasing the risk of cardiac problems. It is estimated that in the year 2000, 171 million people had diabetes, and this is expected to double by year 2030. Conventionally, insulin-dependant diabetes mellitus is treated with exogenous insulin and non insulin-dependant diabetes mellitus with synthetic oral hypoglycemic agents like sulphonylureas and biguanides. However the hormone fails as a curative agent for complications of diabetes and synthetic oral drugs produce adverse health effects. Different medicinal systems are using the active plant constituents, which discovered as natural hypoglycemic medicine, came from the virtue of traditional knowledge. Herbal drugs are considered free from side effects than synthetic one. They are less toxic, relatively cheap and popular. In India, medicinal plants have been used as natural medicine since the days of Vedic glory. Many of these medicinal plants and herbs are part of our diet as spices, vegetables and fruits. Historically, in 'Atharva-Veda' (about 200 B. C.) description of medicinal plants was made under a separate chapter 'Ayurveda'. Sushruta (about 400 B. C.) compiled classification of 700 herbal drugs under 37 classes in 'Sushruta Samhita' (A compendium of ancient Indian surgery). Charak (about 600 B. C.) made the scientific classification of herbal drugs based on remedial properties in his renowned treatise 'Charaka Samhita' (A compendium of general medicine). In which he described 50 classes of herbal remedies comprising 500 crude drugs. The medicinal values of plants have been tested by trial and error method for a long time by different workers. Even today great opportunities are still open for scientific investigations of herbal medicines for cure of diabetes and its complications.

6

Sustainable Use of Medicinal Plants

Wild plants have been an important component of healthcare throughout human history. Medicinal plants continue to make important contributions to healthcare and livelihoods, and were recently identified by FAO as being among the most valuable non-wood forest products (FAO, 1999). Unfortunately, harvests to meet the demand for a growing number of medicinal species are in many cases exceeding sustainable levels. Wild medicinal plant populations and the benefits derived therefrom are coming under threat as a result.

More effective co-operation among the variety of institutions concerned with the use and trade of medicinal plants, including those from the healthcare, conservation, development and commercial sectors, is required to ensure the conservation of biodiversity and continued availability of medicinal resources.

MEDICINAL PLANTS AND HEALTH

Medicinal plants underpin healthcare practices across the globe. Much of the world's population depends on traditional medicine to meet daily health requirements, especially within developing countries. Traditional medicine in turn relies heavily on medicinal plants. Reliance on natural medicinal resources can be attributed to cultural preferences as well as to the high cost and inaccessibility of western medicine.

Use of plant-based remedies is also widespread in many industrialised countries. Herbal remedies are made directly from plant materials, and numerous pharmaceutical products are based on or derived from plant compounds. Similarly, cosmetics and other household products may contain plants of medicinal or therapeutic value. The use of medicinal plants for healthcare is believed to be increasing throughout much of the world, *e.g.* in Africa (Cunningham, 1993; Marshall, 1998), China (He and Sheng, 1997), Europe (Lange, 1998) and North America (Brevoort, 1998).

Commercial Trade in Medicinal Plants

The large and growing demand for plant-based medicines and changing population patterns have prompted a growing domestic and international trade in medicinal plants. The following information from Lange (1997, 1998) gives an indication of the scale of the trade.

According to Customs data, approximately 440 000 t of medicinal and aromatic plants were traded internationally in 1996, with a reported value of USD1.3 billion. Hong Kong, Japan and Germany were the largest importers during 1994 and 1995, the United States being the third largest importer overall during the period 1992 to 1996. Approximately 60% of imports into Germany in 1996 originated from non-European countries, with exports from Asia dominating the trade, followed by exports from Africa. China was also by far the largest exporter of medicinal and aromatic plants to world markets during the mid-1990s, with average exports topping 140 000 t from 1992 to 1996. The second largest exporter was India, with export volumes averaging approximately 36 000 t during this period.

A wide diversity of medicinal plant species are used and traded for medicinal purposes. A recent TRAFFIC 1 study of the European medicinal plant trade (Lange, 1998) estimates that over 2000 medicinal and aromatic plant species are used commercially in Europe, of which 1200 to 1300 are native. Approximately 90% of the European species are collected from the wild, with eastern Europe and the Mediterranean regions being the main suppliers (Lange, 1998). In India it has been estimated that approximately 7500 species are used for medicinal and veterinary purposes (Uniyal et al., 2000). Over 10,000 species are used medicinally in China (He and Cheng, 1991), with 1,000 species commonly used in medicinal preparations, of which 80% are wild-collected (He and Sheng, 1997).

Harvest of medicinal plants to supply domestic and foreign markets provides an important source of cash income in many countries. In Nepal, for example, Olsen (1998, cited in Olsen, 1999) has estimated that 470 000 households are engaged in commercial collection of medicinal plants. Several publications in the FAO Non-Wood Forest Product Series have drawn attention to the current and potential role of medicinal plants in economic development.

Declines in Medicinal Plant Populations

There is growing evidence that the populations of many medicinal plant species are declining in the wild. These declines are the result of several factors, key among them being habitat degradation and expanding harvests. TRAFFIC's study of the European medicinal plant trade identified approximately 150 European species reported to be threatened in at least one

European country (Lange, 1998); a TRAFFIC study in East/Southern Africa identified approximately 100 species of conservation concern in one or more countries (Marshall, 1998). Reviews of the status of medicinal plant species according to the 'Red List' (threat) criteria of IUCN-The World Conservation Union in three regions of India identified approximately 70 species considered at risk (Anon., 1998).

Fourteen species have been included in the Appendices of the Convention on International Trade in Endangered Species of Wild Fauna and Flora (CITES) owing to concern that they might be threatened unless international trade is subject to specific controls.

A MULTI-SECTORAL CHALLENGE

A variety of individuals and institutions have an interest in securing the future of medicinal plant species both because of the direct benefits they provide and in the wider context of biodiversity conservation. These range from local collectors, healers and communities to national governments, multi-national corporations, non-governmental organisations and international treaty bodies. Areas of concern include the role of medicinal plants in healthcare (both local and national) and development, biodiversity conservation, the use of traditional knowledge, intellectual property rights and benefit sharing, marketing and trade.

Individuals acting within different sectors are frequently unaware of the shared and/or conflicting interests and motivations of other sectors. In some cases, this can lead to different sectors unnecessarily working at cross-purposes. For example, government agencies charged with species conservation may be unaware of the importance accorded medicinal plants by health agencies. Similarly, health agencies may be unaware of the status of certain species in the wild. The former may seek to restrict use and trade of specific species, while the latter seeks to expand it.

In many cases, the long-term interests sought by different sectors might be better served through increased information sharing, dialogue and cooperation. For example, efforts to promote commercial trade of medicinal plants as a basis for economic development would benefit from greater knowledge of species biology and market dynamics. Efforts to ensure the conservation of medicinal plant species and their availability for healthcare would similarly benefit from such knowledge. Policies intended to support these and/or other objectives similarly seem more likely to succeed if the full range of stake-holder perspectives and interests are understood and taken into account.

The need for more effective cross-sector collaboration to address medicinal plant conservation issues was first brought to world attention by the

International Consultation on the Conservation of Medicinal Plants, convened by the World Wide Fund for Nature (WWF), IUCN and the World Health Organisation in Chiang Mai, Thailand, in 1988. This message was reiterated a decade later during the international conference Medicinal Plants for Survival, hosted by the Foundation for Revitalization of Local Health Traditions in Bangalore, India in 1998. More recently, 20 participants at the symposium Medicinal Utilisation of Wild Species signed a 'Joint Declaration for the Health of People and Nature', which emphasises the need to address conservation concerns in a multi-disciplinary and collaborative manner. Signatories include representatives of the phytopharmaceutical industry, practitioners' associations and conservation organisations. The depository for the Joint Declaration is WWF Germany, who organised the symposium with TRAFFIC Europe—Germany, and, who, with TRAFFIC, is working to encourage and monitor the Declaration's transformation from words into actions.

These and other initiatives indicate the potential for more and more effective cooperation among individuals and institutions concerned with the use, trade and conservation of medicinal plants. Additional effort needs to be invested in putting these good intentions into practice in order to secure the future of medicinal plant populations and the benefits they provide.

DEVELOPING THE MEDICINAL PLANTS

The medicinal properties of plant species have made an outstanding contribution in the origin and evolution of many traditional herbal therapies. These traditional knowledge systems have started to disappear with the passage of time due to scarcity of written documents and relatively low income in these traditions.

Over the past few years, however, the medicinal plants have regained a wide recognition due to an escalating faith in herbal medicine in view of its lesser side effects compared to allopathic medicine in addition the necessity of meeting the requirements of medicine for an increasing human population. Through the realization of the continuous erosion of traditional knowledge of plants used for medicine in the past and the renewed interest at the present time, a need existed to review this valuable knowledge of medicinal plants with the purpose of developing medicinal plants sectors across the different states in India. Our major objectives therefore were to explore the potential in medicinal plants resources, to understand the challenges and opportunities with the medicinal plants sector, and also to suggest recommendations based upon the present state of knowledge for the establishment and smooth functioning of the medicinal plants sector along with improving the living standards of the underprivileged communities.

The review reveals that northern India harbours a rich diversity of valuable medicinal plants, and attempts are being made at different levels for sustainable utilization of this resource in order to develop the medicinal plants sector.

Background

Forests have played key roles in the lives of people living in both mountains and lowland areas by supplying fresh water and oxygen as well as providing a diversity of valuable forest products for food and medicine. The age-old traditional values attached with the various forest types and the varieties of forest products (*i.e.*, medicinal plants) have gained tremendous importance in the present century.

Furthermore, the cosmetic industries are increasingly using natural ingredients in their products, and these natural ingredients include extracts of several medicinal plants. India and China are two of the largest countries in Asia, which have the richest arrays of registered and relatively well-known medicinal plants. Since the Indian subcontinent is well known for its diversity of forest products and the age-old healthcare traditions, there is an urgent need to establish these traditional values in both the national and international perspectives realizing the ongoing developmental trends in traditional knowledge.

Apart from health care, medicinal plants are mainly the alternate income-generating source of underprivileged communities; therefore, strengthening this sector may benefit and improve the living standard of poor people. A great deal of traditional knowledge of the use of various plant species is still intact with the indigenous people, and this fact is especially relevant with the mountainous areas such as the Himalaya due to less accessibility of terrain and comparatively slow rate of development.

The ongoing growing recognition of medicinal plants is due to several reasons, including escalating faith in herbal medicine. Allopathic medicine may cure a wide range of diseases; however, its high prices and side-effects are causing many people to return to herbal medicines which have fewer side effects.

The instant rising demand of plant-based drugs is unfortunately creating heavy pressure on some selected high-value medicinal plant populations in the wild due to over-harvesting. Several of these medicinal plant species have slow growth rates, low population densities, and narrow geographic ranges; therefore they are more prone to extinction. Conversely, because information on the use of plant species for therapeutic purpose has been passed from one generation to the next through oral tradition, this knowledge of therapeutic plants has started to decline and become obsolete through the lack of recognition by younger generations as a result of a shift in attitude and ongoing socio-economic changes.

Furthermore, the indigenous knowledge on the use of lesser-known medicinal plants is also rapidly declining. Through the realization of the continuous erosion in the traditional knowledge of many valuable plants for medicine in the past and the renewal interest currently, the need existed to review the valuable knowledge with the expectation of developing the medicinal plants sector.

The present paper is therefore concerned with the following major objectives: (1) discovering the role, value, diversity and potential in medicinal plants resources, (2) assessing various aspects of medicinal plant sector, which includes challenges and opportunities, and (3) suggesting recommendations based on existing information for the benefit and development of medicinal plants sector in northern India.

Use and Diversity in Medicinal Plants

In India, of the 17,000 species of higher plants, 7500 are known for medicinal uses. This proportion of medicinal plants is the highest proportion of plants known for their medical purposes in any country of the world for the existing flora of that respective country. Ayurveda, the oldest medical system in Indian sub-continent, has alone reported approximately 2000 medicinal plant species, followed by Siddha and Unani. The Charak Samhita, an age-old written document on herbal therapy, reports on the production of 340 herbal drugs and their indigenous uses. Currently, approximately 25% of drugs are derived from plants, and many others are synthetic analogues built on prototype compounds isolated from plant species in modern pharmacopoeia.

The northern part of India harbours a great diversity of medicinal plants because of the majestic Himalayan range. So far about 8000 species of angiosperms, 44 species of gymnosperms and 600 species of pteridophytes have been reported in the Indian Himalaya, of these 1748 species are known as medicinal plants. The maximum medicinal plants (1717 species) have been reported around the 1800 m elevation range. On the regional scale, the maximum species of medicinal plants have been reported from Uttaranchal, followed by Sikkim and North Bengal. The trans-Himalaya sustains about 337 species of medicinal plants, which is low compared to other areas of the Himalaya due to the distinct geography and ecological marginal conditions.

Several plant species are endemic to the Himalayan region. Out of total known number of higher plants from India, approximately 46% are endemic to the Himalaya. Of the total medicinal plant species, sixty-two species of medicinal plants are endemic to the Himalaya and 208 extend their distribution to the adjacent areas, and are therefore classified as near endemic. Over 200 species of Himalayan medicinal plants are consumed raw, roasted, boiled, fried, cooked, or they are used in the form of oil, spices, jams or pickles.

The indigenous communities use some medicinal plant species as a source of food, fodder, timber as well as various other ethnobotanical purposes. For example, apart from the use of Myrica esculenta and Terminalia bellirica as medicines, the fruits of these species are edible, the leaves are used for fodder and the wood is used for fuel. Approximately 81 species of Himalayan medicinal plants are known to be used for the extraction of oil. Of the total 675 species of Himalayan wild edibles, 171 are used for the treatment of diseases. The crop plants diversity is also a source of traditional medicine .

Apart from the human use, animal husbandry uses many plant species as its primary source of healthcare in northern India. The reliance on medicinal plants is also due to cultural preferences. Medicinal plants have strong acceptance in religious activities of north Indian native communities, who worship the plants in the form of various gods, goddesses and minor deities. Origanum vulgare, Saussurea obvallata, Ocimum sanctum, Cedrus deodara, Cynodon dactylon, Aegle marmelos, Juniperus communis, Musa paradissica, Nardostachys grandiflora, Zanthoxylum armatum, Ficus benghalensis, and Ficus religiosa are examples of the medicinal plants highly used for medicinal as well as a religious purposes by the Hindus in northern India.

The Buddhist community in northern India regards Terminalia chebula as an important medicine as well as sacred fruit. It has been stated long ago that the therapeutic potency of medicinal plants is more effective and better suited to a person of a particular region or culture in which the plant is naturally growing. This idea has given a way to the development of a new drug for heart patients of specific ethnic groups in African countries .

INDUSTRY ROLES IN MEDICINAL PLANT CONSERVATION

This is the story of one company's efforts to source its herbal ingredients from sustainable sources, according to its own account. Pukka Herbs, founded in the UK in 1999, imports plant materials from India and Sri Lanka for the manufacture of ayurvedic preparations. In an interview with Alan Hamilton of Plantlife International, Sebastian Pole, co-founder of Pukka Herbs, emphasised his company's interest in providing high quality health-giving products. Sebastian believes that organic production can be a key to such quality assurance. As with ecological sustainability, verification of organic status requires traceability back to the source areas of the plants, so that Pukka Herbs has a prima-facie motivation to establish traceability.

Pukka Herbs does not buy raw plant materials directly from individual farmers or collectors (which would be a hard task for all but the smallest manufacturers), but does have close relationships with producer companies that work closely with farmers. Pukka does try to restrain the length of its supply chains (which tend to be extensive in the herbal business). Long supply chains, with many intermediate traders between producers and manufacturers, compound the difficulties of tracing the movements of plant materials. They make it difficult for manufacturers to verify that adequate 'production quality' has been achieved for any of the quality categories in which they might be interested - ecological sustainability, product quality (such as organic) and fair trade.

A maximum of three trade links separates Pukka Herbs from the producers of the medicinal plants and usually only two. Pukka purchases plant materials from exporting companies in India and Sri Lanka, that either buy these materials directly from the producers or else buy them from intermediate companies that themselves are directly connected.

EXPORTING COMPANY—PUKKA HERBS

Pukka's ability to achieve traceability for its raw materials, as well as required standards of organic production, has been recognised by the Soil Association, with Pukka's products certified as organic to EU and US standards (the latter under the National Organic Programme). Field certification was by the certifiers SKAL and ECOCERT, their certification being passed on to the Soil Association through recognition of standards' equivalence. Certification was to the normal organic standard of the Soil Association (used mainly for cultivated plants) and not to according to its Organic Wild Crafting Standard, which has more stringent sustainability requirements relating specifically to wild plants.

Principles of 'Production Quality' and their Sharing

Pukka's relationships with a few exporting companies in India and Sri Lanka are central to its business. These exporters are reported by Pukka Herbs to be ecologically and ethically minded agricultural companies that purchase crops from farmers, as well as providing them with training, advice, seeds and fair-trade relationships. Pukka's trading partners were not involved in some of the more specialised Ayurvedic medicinal plants prior to their relationships with Pukka.

Pukka Herbs is committed through its business principles to high quality in three aspects of production: high quality ingredients from the medicinal perspective, ecological sustainability and fair trade. As regards sustainability, Pukka Herbs has its own working document on standards and guidelines to guide its efforts to achieving sustainable harvest. This document is based closely on the standards of the Soil Association, covering both cultivated and wild plants. Special emphasis is placed on the need for management systems for wild plants to be adaptive, allowing rapid and appropriate response to changing circumstances.

The social agenda of Pukka Herbs aims to enhance the livelihoods of the producers of the medicinal plants through enhancing their autonomy. Specific objectives are to develop long-term relationships with the producers (including for the promotion of sustainable production practices and long-term planning), the payment of premium prices that include the cost of sustainable production, the provision of technical assistance and advice, the encouragement or strengthening of community groups for self-empowerment, and the promotion of local markets for organic production (to spread the risks to the producers, so that they are not uniquely bound to Pukka Herbs for market access).

Pukka's business principles must be shared by its business partners in India and Sri Lanka, if they are to be carried into effect. It is these business partners that can give field reality to Pukka's own objectives, which, in the sustainability arena, include the establishment of systems of sustainable harvesting for wild plants, the training of farmers in organic agriculture and assistance for the establishment of nurseries (whether to produce seedlings for field crops or for enrichment planting in the wild).

Pukka Herbs has developed memoranda of understanding (MOU) with its business partners regarding intentions, aspirations and operating standards, covering:

- Organic farming standards
- Commitment to fair trade
- Medicinal plant quality
- Processing standards
- Attainment of Good Agricultural Practice (GAP) and Good Manufacturing Practice (GMP).

Pukka Herbs undertakes an annual exercise in relationship building, technical auditing and quality inspection at randomly selected growing and processing areas to ensure that the terms of the MOU are being met. Relationships are being built 'inclusively', recognising that current practices are not perfect, but rather 'work-in-progress'. The company reports that, with a willingness to learn and a spirit of co-operation, steady progress is proving possible, year-by-year.

The Forest Gardens

Most of the plant materials purchased by Pukka Herbs are actually derived from field crops, rather than wild plants. Of course, there are benefits for plant conservation from organic agriculture, but the parts of Pukka's business most strongly relevant to wider plant conservation are two cases of harvesting wild or semi-wild plants in Sri Lanka. One of these involves the production of medicinal plants in 'forest gardens' and the other the collection of medicinal plants from natural habitats. The exceptional plant conservation interests here are the possibilities of conserving natural populations of plants with their genetic diversity and ecological connections, and opportunities to provide incentives for the conservation of natural or semi-natural habitats containing a diversity of plants.

The forest (or home) gardens of Sri Lanka are famous for their plant diversity, with a total of more than 400, mostly indigenous, species of woody plants recorded. These gardens are tended patches of vegetation of intermediate status between fully wild and fully domesticated. Found in all climatic parts of the island - from the wet rainforest regions of the southwest and centre to the drier wooded savannas of the north and east- the forest gardens of Sri Lanka are economically important to the nation, being the source of 41 per cent of its saw-logs and 26 per cent of its biofuel (Ariyadasa 2002; FSMP 1995). They contain a large number of medicinal plants, including the scrambler Asparagus racemosus, the small shrub Munronia pinnata, the large climbers Coscinum fenestratum and Tinospora cordifolia, and the trees Strychnos nux-vomica and Syzygium cumini.

For the purposes of judging ecological sustainability, a choice must be made for the forest gardens as whether to regard them as cultivated or wild. Sustainability can be judged very differently in the two cases. As typically defined, sustainable agriculture refers to a quite different set of required criteria to sustainability for a wild plant resource. Sustainable agriculture primarily requires maintenance of the basic quality of the land, particularly as regards the quality of the soil, and there is no special need for continuing production of any particular crop in a particular field. In contrast, sustainability with reference to a wild plant resource typically requires that the resource re-grows - most stringently defined as reforming at a rate at least as fast as its rate of extraction. For the purposes of resource management (as opposed to certification requirements), Pukka Herbs decided to regard the forest gardens as wild rather than cultivated (an excellent decision from the wider plant conservation perspective). There then ensued questions about how to ensure that the management and harvesting of medicinal plants in these gardens conformed to standards required for sustainability.

Developing Management Systems for the Forest Gardens

Garden ownership, allowable off-take and enrichment planting were among matters that required addressing to establish satisfactory systems of garden management for sustainability. On ownership, it is widely recognised that a key requirement for proper management of a natural resource is security of rights over its use. For example, the Organic Wild Crafting Standard of the Soil Association requires the designation of a responsible manager for each production area. When Pukka Herbs turned its attention to the forest gardens, it discovered that many were not legally registered, creating an obstacle for certification and possibly also for good management.

A lack of legal title for land or plant resources is a common condition in many developing countries and does not necessarily imply a lack of proper management. Customary rules that are publicly respected can also convey the necessary degree of recognised authority. However, in this case, Pukka Herbs, in association with a producing partner (Lanka Organics), considered it necessary to devote considerable effort to getting the land registered, so that the farmers then legally owned the land and their produce could be certified as organic.

The approach taken to setting levels of off-take for the forest gardens was to request officers from the Forest Department to set annual quotas for each species to be harvested, based on discussions with the producer companies and the farmers, and judgements of the levels at which they could be sustainably harvested in particular gardens. These estimates were rule-of-thumb assessments, based on fairly casual observations of the abundance of the species and general knowledge of their ecologies.

No precise measurements were made of the amounts of the species present or of their rates of regeneration or re-growth. In view of the many uncertainties, the levels of allowable off-take were set conservatively, following the precautionary principle. The Forest Department undertakes annual inspections to verify adherence to the set harvesting levels.

The owners of the forest gardens were encouraged to establish small nurseries of some valuable medicinal plants to produce seedlings for enrichment planting. Criteria for species selection included appropriateness for growing in particular climatic regions, saleability and price. Only local and indigenous species were used, examples including Phyllanthus emblica, Piper longum and Tinospora cordifolia.

Harvesting Medicinal Plants from Natural Habitats

The other example of special relevance for wider plant conservation is also in Sri Lanka and concerns the harvesting of medicinal plants in an area of natural forest. The site, near the town of Bibile in the 'intermediate' climatic zone of Sri Lanka, had earlier been chosen as one of five representative Medicinal Plant Conservation Areas (MPCA) in Sri Lanka by a project of the World Conservation Union (IUCN).

The MPCA at Bibile consists of a core forested area and a surrounding zone with farms. During its period of involvement, the IUCN project started to develop systems of sustainable harvesting for medicinal plants in buffer zones of the forest, as well as inaugurating a medicinal plant demonstration garden and involving around 50 local farmers in medicinal plant production.

However, linkages to the market were poor and, as its project came to an end, IUCN requested Lanka Organics in partnership with Pukka Herbs to see whether it could assist the initiatives that it had started to continue and be developed. As a consequence, Lanka Organics, a local business associate of Pukka, has helped some local farmers to achieve certified organic production of medicinal plants and assisted in the development of sustainable harvesting systems for a few species of wild medicinal trees.

The species selected for sustainable wild production are all plants in which it is the fruits that are required by the medicinal trade, making over-harvesting less of a worry than it would be, for example, if it was roots that were needed. They include Phyllanthus emblica, Terminalia cheluba and T. bellirica.

Possible Future Steps

This case study raises questions about how best to develop practical management and harvest guidelines for each species of medicinal plant harvested from natural vegetation at a particular location. Detailed information on the abundance, regeneration and re-growth rates of harvested species has either been unavailable or not of practical use, either in the case of the forest gardens or at Bibile.

Rather, the approach used has been to set conservative limits to the types or amounts of products allowed for harvest, based on rule-of-thumb estimates of species abundance and recovery rates, and the likely damage likely to be incurred to the plants through collection. Species- and site-specific collection guidelines may be further developed.

A related issue is about how far quantitative rigour is required or possible for the certification of wild-collected medicinal plants as sustainable. In the present case, organic certification was achieved without the need for a high degree of quantitative rigour in resource assessment or monitoring. Conservation organisations have recently been giving increased thought to certification schemes for sustainability, sometimes requiring many measurements and observations on the status of medicinal species and their habitats to achieve certification.

On the other hand, the herbal and botanical sectors are beset with increasing amounts of regulations, compliance with which can be especially difficult for smaller companies, and there are also the challenges of finding finance and expertise required for sophisticated schemes. The challenge of developing workable systems for certifying sustainable wild collection remains.

MEDICINAL PLANTS

Traditional medicines are used by about 60 per cent of the world's population. These are not only used for primary health care not just in rural areas in developing countries, but also in developed countries as well where modern medicines are predominantly used. While the traditional medicines are derived from medicinal plants, minerals, and organic matter, the herbal drugs are prepared from medicinal plants only.

Use of plants as a source of medicine has been inherited and is an important component of the health care system in India. In the Indian systems of medicine, most practitioners formulate and dispense their own recipes, hence this requires proper documentation and research.

In western world also, the use of herbal medicines is steadily growing with approximately 40 per cent of population reporting use of herb to treat medical illnesses within the past year. Public, academic and government interest in traditional medicines is growing exponentially due to the increased incidence of the adverse drug reactions and economic burden of the modern system of medicine.

There are about 45,000 plant species in India, with concentrated hotspots in the region of Eastern Himalayas, Western Ghats and Andaman & Nicobar Island. The officially documented plants with medicinal potential are 3000 but traditional practitioners use more than 6000. India is the largest producer of medicinal herbs and is appropriately called the botanical garden of the world.

There are currently about 250 000 registered medical practitioners of the Ayurvedic system (total for all traditional systems: approximately 291 000), as compared to about 700,000 of the modern medicine system. In rural India, 70 per cent of the population is dependent on the traditional system of medicine, the Ayurveda.

MEDICINAL PLANTS—INDUSTRIAL PROFILES

Which well known plant never touches the ground, does not follow a 12-month vegetation cycle, stays green year round, blooms in the winter, and sells predominately in December? The answer, of course, is mistletoe. Current research questions the efficacy of this highly controversial plant. "Rejected by clinical oncologists but used by practitioners and cancer patients, it is applied as a remedy to treat a broad spectrum of different diseases, such as epilepsy, diabetes, hypertension, arthrosis, hepatitis, HIV infection, labour pains, and cancer."

Now a new book on the therapeutic uses and industrial applications of Viscum has been published. Rarely mentioned in traditional books on herbal medicine mistletoe research remains questionable. Because the "extracts may exert different effects than purified substances" individual immune responses vary greatly. There is a great need for further investigation. Currently no clinical data are available documenting long-term therapy treatment.

Whether the extracts of Viscum become a major player in the fight against cancer, this book makes for provocative reading. Researchers in pharmacognosy and phystochemistry will find this book documented with references to hundreds of research articles invaluable. While most articles feature the European point of view, there is one article from Japan and another from South Africa. Although none of the articles originate from the United States, American research is well represented in the bibliographies, as are traditional Chinese uses for this herb.

Responding to the increased demand for information on medicinal and aromatic plants this fascinating look at this highly controversial plant is the 16th volume in the series Medicinal and Aromatic Plants Industrial Profiles. This series brings together articles scattered through a variety of sources, is international in scope, and includes many little known sources. Each article is well documented and is introduced by the editor Arndt Bussing, head of the Department of Applied Immunology at the foundation Krebsforschung Herdecke, University of Witten/Herdecke. Mistletoe: the Genus Viscum is illustrated with colour photographs of the plant, line drawings, and chemical structures. With few exceptions most references are current, dating from 1990 to 2000.

While this book would be of interest to scientists in botany, agriculture, and phytochemistry, those working in alternative medicine, pharmaceutical, and health sciences should find it of greater interest. Recommended for academic and research libraries.

NEW SUPPORT FOR MEDICINAL PLANTS

Aspirin, ginseng tea, Aloe lotions and gels are simple healthcare remedies used in many parts of the world to treat a variety of illnesses. They all also have a common beginning: wild plants. Aspirin, for instance, owes its origins to the willow tree.

Hippocrates used powder extracted from willow bark to treat pain and reduce fever in the fifth century BC. Over 2000 years later, the chemical compound salicin was isolated from willow bark, the precursor to the active compound found in modern aspirin. Today, it is estimated that more than 80 billion aspirin tablets are used each year in the USA alone. Unlike aspirin, ginseng tea, used to improve vital energy and slow aging, is still produced from the raw product: ginseng roots. However, much of the ginseng in trade is cultivated, as is all of the aloe vera gel found in skin-care products and health drinks.

Less well known are the tens and perhaps hundreds of thousands of other medicinal plant species used around the world, some of which, like willow trees, have been recognised for their healing properties for thousands of years.

These plants form the basis of health care systems throughout much of the developing world, a source of new compounds on which to base new pharmaceutical products, and a major component of the burgeoning markets for herbal health care remedies and natural products. They also provide a source of income for growers, traders, collectors and manufacturers of plant-based medicines.

In this dual role as a source of healthcare and income, medicinal plants make an important contribution to the larger development process. Unfortunately, however, some plant species of medicinal value are already in short supply, which poses a threat to human welfare and the wild species themselves. Immediate actions are therefore required to ensure harvest and trade of medicinal plant species are conducted sustainably.

TRAFFIC has been working on the medicinal plant trade for many years, including collaboration with important partners such as the IUCN/SSC Medicinal Plant Specialist Group.

Germany's Federal Ministry for Economic Cooperation and Development (Bundesministerium fur wirtschaftliche Zusammenarbeit, more commonly known as BMZ) is supporting a suite of new actions by TRAFFIC. Through a Funds in Trust Agreement with WWF International, BMZ has pledged DM1 million (US$560 000) to the TRAFFIC Network's medicinal plant work during 1998-2000. Much of the funding is directed toward regionally focused work in East Asia, the Indian subcontinent and South America.

In addition, BMZ is supporting efforts to build and/or strengthen links with others working on medicinal plant trade issues. It aims to enhance the communication of TRAFFIC's research results to those who need it, from traditional medicine communities to policy makers.

The regional work to be undertaken through BMZ support is as diverse as the medicinal plant trade itself, with each region home to different, but in the case of India and East Asia, overlapping, medicinal traditions.

East Asia

The major traditional medicine systems in this region are derived from traditional Chinese medicine (TCM), which has a history of several thousand years and is well-documented.

Although international attention has been drawn to the use of animal species such as rhinoceros and Tiger in TCM, animal ingredients actually make up less than 20% of those used in TCM. TCM is largely a plant-based medicinal system. It is believed that as many as 1000 plant species are in use for TCM in China and that about 80 per cent of them are taken from the wild. An initial TRAFFIC East Asia study in Hong Kong in 1995/96 revealed a massive trade involving a number of threatened plant species: of the 388 plant species listed in the China Plant Red Data Book, 69 were found to be used in TCM, and 22 of these were in common use.

Through work supported by BMZ, TRAFFIC East Asia seeks to promote the security and conservation of wild plant resources used in traditional medicine in East Asia to support basic health care needs. TRAFFIC East Asia will convene a series of meetings to promote dialogue and understanding of the links between conservation and medicinal security issues among producers, regulators and medicinal communities.

Other activities planned include the compilation of an overview of the nature of and trends in medicinal plant harvest, propagation and trade in East Asia; identifying species at risk; and reviewing national legislation and policies relevant to production, supply and conservation of medicinal plants. Work will also be undertaken to help build capacity within governments and TCM communities to implement any needed trade controls.

The Indian subcontinent

The Himalayas provide more than a meeting point for China and the Indian subcontinent. They also provide a huge variety and volume of medicinal plants used in TCM, Tibetan medicine, and Ayurved. Like TCM, Ayurved has a long history (over 3000 years), is well-documented, and is widely used both locally and in Asian communities established in other parts of the world. There are also a large number of localised traditional medicine systems.

Harvest of native plants to supply India's own healthcare needs and a growing export market provides an important source of income for local communities. However, demand for plant materials is huge and growing, while many of the region's medicinal plant resources are dwindling.

Recent reviews applying IUCN threat criteria found that a significant number of medicinal plant species are threatened or endangered within India. Large quantities of raw medicinal plant materials are also imported into India from neighbouring countries and exported to overseas markets.

A number of organizations within India are concerned with maintaining India's traditional medicine systems. In addition, there is a widespread development network, an established pharmaceutical industry and a wealth of botanical experts in the country. Until now, however, there has been little effort to document the volume and impact of national or international trade in India's medicinal plants.

TRAFFIC India is already well on its way toward establishing working relationships with key stake-holders such as those above and government personnel and toward collecting information required if plants in trade are to be managed on a sustainable basis.

A key challenge within India will be to inform these and other stake-holders of the nature and impact of the medicinal plant trade, and to facilitate their co-operation in developing and implementing measures that will secure the conservation of medicinal plants. Original research will be combined with meetings and workshops to discuss findings and develop workable solutions to any problems identified.

South America

In contrast to East Asia and India, South America's traditional medicine practices are far more localised, with neither the geographic extent or the written texts that characterise TCM and Ayurved. As a result, an important first step is to study and describe the medicinal plant trade in the region, to identify commonly used species, and to begin the process of identifying whether any species are at risk.

Preliminary research in 1996 and 1997 by TRAFFIC International's South America Plants Officer confirmed that, as in Asia, medicinal plants are important components of local health care, are in some cases used unsustainably, and are exported as well as used locally.

BMZ funding is supporting the completion of a regional overview of the medicinal plant trade as well as more detailed studies of individual species in trade, existing trade controls, and the potential role of regional and international treaties in this region. Two species already identified for further research are Cat's Claw Uncaria tomentosa and Dragon's Blood Croton lechleri.

The results of this research will be shared with governments, traditional healthcare associations and relevant agencies to further raise the profile of medicinal plant trade issues and stimulate discussion and actions necessary to ensure more effective management.

MEDICINAL PLANTS AND CITES

The Challenge of Sustainable Harvest

Plants of medicinal value originate from all over the world. Harvest occurs for both local and international use. A growing problem, which is compounded by global population growth and increased demand for raw materials, is over-exploitation of these important resources. The vast majority of medicinal plants used in traditional medical systems and natural products industries are collected from the wild. While propagation occurs for a few species such as American Ginseng Panax quinquefolius and Kuth Saussurea costus, propagation is generally limited due to the expense and time periods required for plants to reach salable size. Harvest and trade can be an important source of income for rural peoples. Regrettably, unsustainable harvest is an increasingly common occurrence that threatens not only the future of these species, but also the livelihoods and health status of people throughout the world.

The Current Situation

At present an estimated 230 plant species included in CITES are traded for medicinal purposes, or are likely to be traded in the future. Fourteen of these were specifically included in the Appendices expressly because of the need to regulate trade in medicinal material. A further six species, Adonis vernalis, Camptotheca acuminata, Cistanche deserticola, Harpagophytum procumbens, Harpagophytum zeyheri and Panax ginseng, are proposed for inclusion in Appendix II at COP11. The Parties' implementation of the Convention for the species currently included in the Appendices is poor, and is in many cases non-existent. This is surprising, given the importance of these species to the health care of the peoples of these nations, to the livelihoods of the millions who derive income from medicinal plant harvest and trade, and to the industries and consumers who benefit from these resources. Indeed, some Parties have made notable efforts to implement CITES for medicinal plants, such as Germany with the publication of the Checklist of Medicinal and Aromatic Plants and their Trade Names covered by CITES and EU Regulation 2307/97 and Identification Training for Medicinal and Aromatic Plants covered by CITES and EU Regulation 2307/97, and USA with the establishment of a ginseng management programme to monitor wild populations and regulate harvest and commerce.

The Plants Committee has examined the trade through the Medicinal Plant Significant Trade Study, and additional significant plant trade surveys have been undertaken by TRAFFIC. However, these efforts are few in number and although Parties may have taken domestic measures to conserve native plant populations, in general, implementation of the Convention for medicinal plants is unsatisfactory.

Over-exploitation of medicinal plants, and lack of attention to illegal and unsustainable trade, is having serious repercussions around the world. As the global population expands, the demand for medicine increases correspondingly. International trade in medicinal and aromatic plants is already massive, with for example, annual global market imports totalling 440,000 metric tonnes in 1996, at a value of USD 1.3 billion. The medicinal plant trade can make a considerable contribution to the economies of producer countries.

Searching for Solutions

As medicinal plant populations decline, governments, natural resource managers, local communities and a variety of other stake-holders have attempted to address the problem in order to conserve medicinal resources. Efforts have been varied.

For example, these initiatives include: promotion of sustainable harvesting techniques; improvement of marketing and trade opportunities to ensure better management; training in quality control and packaging to reduce wastage and derive higher earnings; increased regulation and control at local, national and international levels; and propagation of medicinal plant species. Increasingly, these efforts are designed taking into consideration the complexity of the medicinal plant issue and the realization that demand will not decrease, hence solutions must factor in the aspect of a continuously increasing trade.

The market for medicinal plants is dynamic and complex. Demand for new natural products, and growing interest in traditional medical systems around the world, means that greater volumes of plant material are required to satisfy the market. Medicinal plants are traded in a variety of forms, for example: raw material such as leaves, bark, and roots, unprocessed broken material such as chips or slices, derivatives and semi-processed or manufactured material such as powders, extracts, tonics, pills, teas and other products, as well as finished pharmaceutical products.

Trade occurs far from the area of production, and processing often takes place in countries other than those where the plants originate. For example, approximately 120,000 metric tonnes of medicinal and aromatic plants were imported into Europe in 1996, and this material came from over 120 countries, 60% of which were African and Asian nations. During this same year, Europe exported about 70,000 metric tonnes of plant material. Understanding the dynamics of the trade in medicinals can be difficult, and although overall volumes and values may be known, species-specific information is not at all comprehensive. The dearth of such data is one reason for the lack of attention countries have directed toward the medicinal plant resource.

Insufficient knowledge about the scope of the trade, in particular at the range state level, has resulted in ineffective implementation of existing regulations and initiatives in producing countries, to the detriment of the resource and those who will depend on it in the years to come. Perhaps most important is that there is little appreciation for the increasingly critical imbalance between supply and demand.

Can CITES Help?

CITES addresses only a small portion of the medicinal plant issue, but it has the potential to help achieve sustainable and legal trade in medicinal resources. Specifically, CITES can do the following:

- identify trends at the species level and on the global level, to highlight critical issues and address them;
- help to make the trade more transparent, by documenting the species and parts in trade, and volumes traded, because this information is necessary for designing and implementing sustainable management plans;
- stimulate cooperation between importing and exporting countries to ensure that trade is conducted in a legal and sustainable manner;

So What is the Problem?

When the trade is so large, and the implications of unsustainable harvest and trade so serious, why is implementation of CITES for medicinal plants unsatisfactory? Some possible explanations include the following:

- Parties are unaware that CITES-listed medicinal plants are in international trade, because of insufficient knowledge about the parts and derivatives that aretraded.
- Regulatory officials responsible for inspection of plant material are unfamiliar with CITES and do not know that certain traded plant species require CITES documentation.
- Plants are frequently afforded less attention than animal species.
- The variety of parts and derivatives in trade is numerous, and the annotations for CITES- listed medicinal plants vary from species to species, therefore it may be difficult for inspectors to keep track of what should be regulated.
- The majority of trade in medicinal and aromatic plants is not regulated by CITES, and therefore CITES-listed species may be accorded a low priority.

Will these Efforts help Medicinal Plants?

At present the sustainability of the medicinal plant trade is on precarious ground. Through CITES, there is an opportunity to promote sustainable harvest and trade. While regulation is only part of the solution, it is an integral part of a strategy that must entail efforts from many sectors and many directions.

Because of the importance of a sustainable trade in medicinal plants, it is entirely appropriate for CITES to collaborate and indeed advise other global bodies that deal directly with human health issues, on the conservation aspect of this problem. With regard to medicinal plants, the objectives of CITES and the CBD are complementary.

Demand for Medicinal Plants in KwaZulu-Natal

Medicinal plants are used extensively by the black population throughout KwaZulu-Natal (KZN), and indeed South Africa. An active trade and market in medicinal plant material occurs in KwaZulu-Natal as a result of:

- a fragmented distribution of medicinal plant species due to the varied land use, topography and climate in the region,
- large spatial concentrations of consumer demand as more than half the province's population is concentrated in two urban centres,
- local extinctions of plants and the need to access more remote plant populations due to intensive harvesting, and
- various socio-economic factors (including culture and accessible health care) which maintain and stimulate demand.

In KwaZulu-Natal over 400 plants are actively traded [Cunningham 1988; McKean 1996] with an estimated trade volume of some 4 300 tonnes per year. As the market is large and dynamic, several market segments have developed in response to the users' demands and the supply of plants. The extent of trade and the market segments are discussed in the following sections.

Quantity and Trends in Consumer Demand

A survey of several Durban City medical clinics indicated that 53% of the black clinic patients made use of indigenous healers at least once during the previous year, with an average of 3.34 visits in the previous year. The term indigenous healers or medicine is preferred by the author to the more conventional term traditional healers or medicine. The healing practices used, while originating in African culture, are not purely traditional. The practice is dynamic, addressing new illnesses like AIDS, and adopts new technologies and new medicines.

The healers also deal with all manner of urban social problems, which are not traditional. The term indigenous medicine may therefore be more appropriate as it relates to the practices of healing and divination within an indigenous but modem African culture which may not necessarily be traditional.

While respondents asked whether they visited a indigenous healer in the previous year, the survey omitted to ask respondents whether they purchased indigenous medicine without a healer's prescription. As a consequence, the above estimate of indigenous medicine use may be an underestimate. An indication of the extent of self-medication can be obtained from the expressed preference for hygienically packed medicines.

Eighty-four percent of the black clinic patients indicated that they would prefer more hygienically packed indigenous medicines, indicating that 31% of the sample may not have visited an indigenous healer in 1995 but probably make use of indigenous medicine.

Assuming that the clinic sample is representative of the black population in Durban, the total number of users is estimated to be around 2 million people [that is 84% of 2.442 million blacks resident in Durban (Durban Metropolitan Government 19.96)]. This estimate can be considered a conservative minimum level, as 6% of the indigenous healers patients indicated that they did not make use of western clinics, and therefore using the clinic patients as a proxy for the Durban black population may be a slight underestimate.

The Quantity of Plant Material Reported to be Consumed

Basing the quantity demanded on the reported number of times which the population sample visits indigenous healers (3.34 times per annum), it is estimated that between 900 tonnes and 1 500 tonnes of plant material were consumed in Durban in 1995 .

As most of the estimates are based on relatively imprecise data regarding the numbers of market participants, the broad estimates will generally be rounded off to make for easier reading. However, detailed measurements made within the survey will be retained for descriptive accuracy and where calculations are made.

This estimate assumes that the indigenous medicine users not visiting indigenous healers, that is the remaining 31% of users, would use indigenous medicine at the same rate at which healers are visited (3.34 times a year). The estimate of 900 tonnes is derived if 53% of the population is assumed to use medicine at an average mass of 83.3g per use (the average mass of plant material prescribed by healers and shop traders) and the remaining consumers use the medicine at 216.5g per use (the average mass of plant material traded in the street markets). The estimate of 1 500 tonnes is obtained if all 84% of the black population uses medicine at 216.5g per use. This last estimate is likely to be more realistic given the extent of wastage associated with the poor storage of plant material.

The Quantity of Plant Material Reported to be Traded

The shop traders are estimated to trade 340 tonnes per year, with approximately 50% reported to be purchased directly from plant gatherers (170 tonnes) and the remaining 50% purchased from street traders (170 tonnes).

The quantities traded by the healers was problematic to estimate due to the unknown number of healers in the survey area. Various reports [Holdstock

1978; Gelfand 1985; Cunningham 1988] had been made regarding the ratio of indigenous healers to the population but these have not been used for a number of reasons.

Firstly, the mode of operation differs considerably between healers, with some healers being extremely busy whilst others may only practise part-time. Secondly, the various healers' organizations have provided a rough indications of the number of healers which are registered with them, but it has not been possible to obtain membership lists from these groups (in addition, the membership makes no differentiation regarding the nature of the practitioners operation, that is, whether it is either full-time or part-time).

Due to the above problems, estimates are based on the visitation frequency reported by the clinic patients and the average number of patients, which the indigenous healers indicate they may treat per day. Following this approach an estimated 936 tonnes of medicinal plants are traded per year by indigenous healers in Durban.

The indigenous healers reported that they purchase plant material from two sources, approximately 50% from the street markets and 50% directly from plant gatherers. This suggests that approximately 468 tonnes are bought from each group.

This estimate uses an average mass of 216.5 g for a prescribed medicine dosage. This mass is the average mass of street traded products and is believed to be a more appropriate mass than the mass dispensed in traders shops and by healers (an average 83.3 g) for estimating the quantity used by healers. The traded products are generally unprocessed and poorly packaged, with a significant proportion (not quantifiable at present) of the plant material spoiled in the transportation and storage process. The author therefore considers the larger street traded mass to be a more accurate reflection of the quantities which healers will utilise but not necessarily dispense.

Of the plant mass traded in the street markets, an estimated 20% of the trade or 220 tonnes, is reported to be traded between the street traders themselves and not to consumers, healers or shop traders. This implies that of the 1 100 tonnes traded in the market as a whole, only 880 tonnes of plant material is the physical stock of plants entering the street markets in a year. By summing the quantities sold by the various market players to end consumers, it is estimated that some 1 500 tonnes of plant material were sold in the Durban markets in 1996.

This estimate of 1 500 tonnes traded in the market approximates the estimate derived in 4.1.1 regarding the maximum quantity of plant material which may be consumed in Durban given the consumption rates of the clinic patients interviewed. While the two approaches are not entirely independent as both models use a common number in estimating the use associated with healers, there is sufficiently different information in the other sectors which gives confidence to the similarity of estimates.

Potential Provincial and National Consumption Levels

Several studies in different geographic localities throughout South Africa and in different cultural groups have shown that between 58 and 100% of the black population uses indigenous medicine. Holdstock [1978] estimated that between 80 and 85% of the black population in Soweto (a black township in Johannesburg) consumed indigenous medicine. Ellis [1986] found that 100% of a random sample of hospital patients in the Estcourt area (a typical rural population) used indigenous medicine. More recently, a study in peri-urban Bushbuckridge [Mander 1997a] estimated that 58% of the clinic patients used indigenous medicine. However, this estimate is known to be conservative due to the persecution of people suspected of witchcraft in the area, and consequently an unwillingness to admit to the use of indigenous medicine. Assuming that the characteristics of the Durban consumers are representative of the rest of the population in KwaZulu-Natal and South Africa, it is possible to provide a preliminary indication of provincial and national consumption patterns. In KwaZulu-Natal the current population is estimated to be 8.7 million, with the black population comprising 83% of the total population or 7.2 million people [Central Statistical Services 1996]. Assuming that 84% of the black population use indigenous medicine in KwaZulu-Natal, the number of potential users of indigenous medicine could therefore be 6 million people. Based on an average frequency of uses of 3.34 visits/uses per year (this translates to 20 million uses a year), and assuming an average mass of 216.5g per use, then total quantity of medicinal plants used in KwaZulu-Natal could amount to 4 339 tonnes per year.

Similarly, at a national level there are 33 million blacks in South Africa [Central Statistical Services 1996] with an estimated 28 million (84%) users. Using the same visitation rate per year and the mass per use as above, the total national consumption could amount some 90 million uses per year with a mass of 19 500 tonnes of plant material.

Trends in the Use of Indigenous Medicine

The survey of consumer trends at western clinics and at indigenous healers indicated that a large section of the population has not changed their use patterns, with similar percentages indicating both an increase and a decrease in use. There is, however, an overall increase in the use of indigenous medicine. The following figures (4.3 to 4.8) and discussion outline the changes and reasons for change in use frequency cited by healers and clinic patients.

Of the indigenous healers interviewed, 90% believed that the demand for indigenous medicine would remain high. The shop traders shared the same perspective that trade would remain at high levels.

Discussions with market players and observations of the markets in southern Africa (South Africa, Mozambique, Swaziland, Lesotho and Namibia) have pointed to an increase in the demand for medicines [Scott pers. comm. 1996; Maseko pers. comm. 1997]. While the individual consumers surveyed may not have indicated a trend of increasing use, there is common consensus among traders and researchers that there has been an increase in the number of individuals consuming indigenous medicine. This may be the result of the following factors.

The population growth throughout the region is around 2.4% per year [Central Statistics 1996], leading to an increase in the potential number of people who may make use of indigenous medicine. Coupled with this increase, are the accelerated urbanization rates, which increase the competition for resources and services, especially where economic growth lags behind population growth. Indigenous medicines are actively used to reduce competition for employment, housing, and other social resources that are associated with increasing urban competition. Competition in urban areas may also contribute to psychological stress, and indigenous healing and healers are used extensively to treat stress-related illness.

The existence of poverty also fuels the demand for medicinal plants as households are forced to make use of affordable medicine. While consulting a healer may be more expensive than visiting a clinic, medicines bought directly from the street traders are much cheaper than any other forms of health care, and consequently are an important health care option.

Past government policies in South Africa discriminated against indigenous healing, giving it no positive recognition, and generally labelling the activities as primitive and even legislating against witchcraft practices (Suppression of Witchcraft Act). Perceptions are now changing from several quarters, with increasing official and societal recognition. For example, medical aids in South Africa are increasingly accepting claims, by their members, for visits to indigenous healers [Daily News, 14 January 1997], and black people themselves are developing increasing pride in the culture of indigenous healing.

One of the greatest drivers of the demand for indigenous medicine are the widely held views by the black community that certain illnesses are 'cultural' sicknesses which can only be treated by indigenous medicine. In addition, AIDS is rapidly increasing within the South African community, and with little relief from western medicine, healers report that people with AIDS consult them. There are many healers who now advertise that they have a cure for AIDS, promoting the increased use of indigenous medicine.

Apart from the above, the remote geographical location of many large rural populations also promotes the use of indigenous medicine as it is usually the most accessible source of health care, and the most available health care, as western clinics are either far away or visit rural communities only periodically.

In view of the above factors, the local demand for indigenous medicine is unlikely to decline and will probably increase as the population increases.

Apart from growing local demand, there are also indications of a growing international demand. Neighbouring countries (particularly Namibia and Botswana) are increasing their demand for South African medicinal plants due to the greater diversity, reliability of supply and quantities available. The dry environments have relatively low diversities of high value medicinal plants and in addition, the frequent and regular movement of people between southern African states results in considerable exchange in ideas and information, with foreign healers learning to use South African products. In addition, the declining ability of many countries to maintain the importation of synthetic drugs promotes the continued use of indigenous medicines8. International demand for local plant products is also likely to increase with the growing popularity of alternative medicines and natural products in developed countries [Lange 1997].

For example, discussions in 1996 with women from a remote area in western Mali, reported to the author that they did not bother travelling to the local clinic, in this case only a few kilometres away, as the only medicine which the clinic could provide was quinine and aspirin, and good alternatives for these drugs were more easily accessible in the bush close to where they lived.

7

Essential Oil

An essential oil is any concentrated, hydrophobic liquid containing volatile aroma compounds from plants. They are also known as volatile or ethereal oils, or simply as the "oil of" the plant material from which they were extracted, such as oil of clove. The term essential indicates that the oil carries distinctive scent of the plant, not that it is an especially important or fundamental substance. Essential oils do not as a group need to have any specific chemical properties in common, beyond conveying characteristic fragrances. They are not to be confused with essential fatty acids.

Essential oils are generally extracted by distillation. Other processes include expression, or solvent extraction. They are used in perfumes and cosmetics, for flavoring food and drink, and for scenting incense and household cleaning products.

Various essential oils have been used medicinally at different periods in history. Medical applications proposed by those who sell medicinal oils vary from skin treatments to remedies for cancer, and are often based on historical use of these oils for these purposes. Such claims are now subject to regulation in most countries, and have grown correspondingly more vague, to stay within these regulations.

Interest in essential oils has revived in recent decades, with the popularity of aromatherapy, a branch of alternative medicine which claims that the specific aromas carried by essential oils have curative effects. Oils are volatilized or diluted in a carrier oil and used in massage, or burned as incense, for example.

Production

Distillation: Today, most common essential oils, such as lavender, peppermint, and eucalyptus, are distilled. Raw plant material, consisting of the flowers, leaves, wood, bark, roots, seeds, or peel, is put into an alembic (distillation apparatus) over water, As the water is heated the steam passes through the plant material, vaporizing the volatile compounds. The vapours flow through a coil where they condense back to liquid, which is then collected in the receiving vessel.

Most oils are distilled in a single process. One exception is Ylang-ylang (Cananga odorata), which takes 22 hours to complete through a fractional distillation.

The water recondensed from the distillation process is referred to as a hydrosol, hydrolat, herbal distillate or plant water essence, which may be sold as another fragrant product. Popular hydrosols are rose water, lavender water, lemon balm, clary sage and orange blossom water. The use of herbal distillates in cosmetics is increasing. Some plant hydrosols have unpleasant smells and are therefore not sold.

Expression: Most citrus peel oils are usually expressed mechanically, or cold-pressed. Due to the large quantities of oil in citrus peel and the relatively low cost to grow and harvest the raw materials, citrus-fruit oils are cheaper than most other essential oils. Lemon or sweet orange oils that are obtained as by-products of the commercial citrus industry are even cheaper.

Prior to the discovery of distillation, essential oils (EO) were extracted by pressing.

Solvent Extraction: Most flowers contain very little volatile oil to undergo expression and their chemical components are too delicate and easily denatured by the high heat used in steam distillation. Instead, a solvent such as hexane or supercritical carbon dioxide is used to extract the oils. Extracts from hexane and other hydrophobic solvent are called concretes, which is mixture of essential oil, waxes, resins, and other lipophilic (oil soluble) plant material.

Although highly fragrant, concretes contain large quantities of non-fragrant waxes and resins. As such another solvent, often ethyl alcohol, which only dissolves the fragrant low-molecular weight compounds, is used to extract the fragrant oil from the concrete. The alcohol is removed by a second distillation, leaving behind the absolute.

Supercritical carbon dioxide is used as a solvent in supercritical fluid extraction. This method has many benefits, including avoiding petrochemical residues in the product. It does not yield an absolute directly. The supercritical carbon dioxide will extract both the waxes and the essential oils that make up the concrete. Subsequent processing with liquid carbon dioxide, achieved in the same extractor by merely lowering the extraction temperature, will separate the waxes from the essential oils. This lower temperature process prevents the decomposition and denaturing of compounds and provides for a superior product. When the extraction is complete, the pressure is reduced to ambient and the carbon dioxide reverts back to a gas, leaving no residue.

Although supercritical carbon dioxide is also used for making decaffeinated coffee, the actual process is different.

Production Quantities: Estimates of total production of essential oils are difficult to obtain. One estimate, compiled from data in 1989, 1990 and 1994 from various sources gives the following total production, in tonnes, of essential oils for which more than 1,000 tonnes were produced.

Oil	*Tonnes*
Sweet orange	12,000
Mentha arvensis	4,800
Peppermint	3,200
Cedarwood	2,600
Lemon	2,300
Eucalyptus globulus	2,070
Litsea cubeba	2,000
Clove (leaf)	2,000
Spearmint	1,300

SOME OTHER AROMATIC PLANTS

Cucurbits

This group includes cucumber (Cucumis sativus L.), musk-melon (Cucumis melo L.), water-melon (Citrullus vulgaris Schred. Ex Eckl. & Zeyh.), bottle-gourd (Lagenaria siceraria (Mol.) Standl.), bitter-gourd (Momordicac harantia L.), sponge-gourd (Luffa cylindrica (L.) Roem), ridge-gourd (Luffa acutangula Roxb.), snake-gourd (Trichosanthes anguina L.), pointed-gourd (parwal) (Trichosanthes dioica Roxb.), round-gourd (tinda) (Citrullus vulgaris var. Fistulosus Duth. & Full), ash-gourd (Benincasa hispida (Thunb.) Cogn.), pumpkin (Cucurbita moschata Dutch. Ex Poir), summer squash (C. pepo L.), winter squash (C. maxima Duch.) and a number of other crops mostly of trailing habit. They all belong to the family Cucurbitaceae and are grown during summer.

The majority of them are monoecious and a few are dioecious, hermaphrodite and andrmonoecious.

Varieties

Cucumber: 'Japanese Long Green', 'Straight Eight', 'Balam Khira', 'Khira Poona', etc.

Musk-melon: 'Pusa Sharbati', 'Lucknow Safeda', 'Hara Madhum Kutana', 'Durgapur', 'Madhu', 'Arka Jeet', 'Arka Rajhans', etc.

Water-melon: 'Sugar Baby', 'Asahi Yamato', 'Charleston Grey', 'Pusa Badana' (seedless), 'Tetra-2', etc.

Bottle-gourd: 'Pusa Summer Prolific Long', 'Pusa Summer Prolific Round', 'Pusa Meghdut' and 'Pusa Manjari'

Bitter-gourd: 'Pusa Domousmi', 'Kalianpur Baramasi', 'Coimbatore White Long', etc.

Sponge-gourd: 'Pusa Chikni'

Ridge-gourd: 'Pusa Nasdhar', 'Satputia'

Summer squash: 'Early Yellow Prolific', 'Australian Green', 'Butternut', etc.

Winter squash: 'Arkha Suryamukhi'

Tinda: 'Arka Tinda'

Cultivation

The culturalreqs of all the commercially important crops in this group are more or less similar. Cucumber, bottle-gourd, bitter-gourd, pumpkin, sponge-gourd and ridge-gourd can be grown in summer as well as in the rainy season, whereas, musk-melon, water-melon, squashes and tinda grow better only in summer. Winter squash grows well under mild climatic conditions. There are two methods of sowing. Ridges are prepared at proper spacing and after adding manure, a number of seeds are sown on each ridge. In the other method, furrows are made and seeds are sown on the edge either on one or both sides. The spacing from row to row, unless staked, varies from 1-1/2 to 3 m, according to the crop. The distance from plant to plant is kept at 60-90 cm. Approximately 2.5 to 3 kg of seed is required for sowing a hectare of cucumber, musk-melons and water-melon, 4 to 5 kg of seed of bottle-gourd, sponge-gourd and ridge-gourd, and 7 to 8 kg of seed of pumpkin and squashes. The summer crop is sown from January to March and the rainy-season crop in June-July. In the hills, they are sown in April. About 30 tonnes of farmyard manure are added to the soil at the time of preparing the land. For a good yield, 80 kg of nitrogen in two doses and 50 kg each of phosphorus and potassium per hectare should be applied. The average yields per hectare are: bitter-gourd and squashes, 6,000 to 8,000 kg; cucumber and musk-melon, 8,000 to 10,000 kg; water-melon and bottle-gourd, 15,000 to 20,000 kg, and pumpkin, 20,000 to 25,000 kg.

The cucurbits are also grown on the river-beds during summer. Special techniques are followed to get an early crop on the sandy banks of the rivers.

Cucurbitaceous crop are attacked by a number of diseases, of which powdery mildew, downey mildew, Fusarium wilt and virus diseases are of economic importance. Powdery and downey mildews can be controlled by spraying the crop with Karathane or Morestan, or by growing resistant varieties. Red pumpkin beetle and fruit fly are the most important insect pests. Dusting with 1 percent Lindane or a mixture of BHC and DDT control the beetle, but DDT should be dusted with caution, as it may damage the young bit leaves.

Sweet Potato

The sweet potato (Ipomoea batatas (L.) Poir.) is a very important crop in the tropical regions of India. The chief uses of sweet-potato are for human consumption and for the manufacture of starch and alcohol. It contains about 16 per cent starch and about 4 per cent sugar. It belongs to the family Convolvulaceae.

Varieties

'Pusa Suffaid', 'Pusa Lal', 'Pusa Sunheri', 'SP-3', 'SP-9', 'Ranger', 'Bhadrakali', 'Hosur Red', 'Gold Rush', 'Centennial', etc.

Cultivation

Sweet-potato requires a long and warm growing season. It does not stand frost. A moderate proportion of sand in the top soil, with a fairly retentive subsoil, provides ideal condition for its growth. It is grown from sprouts produced from its tuber-like roots and from vine cuttings. In well-prepared nursery-beds, the selected roots are planted 30 cm apart in rows which are spaced 45 cm. The sprouts are cut and planted for further growth in a second nursery. Ultimately, the cuttings from this nursery are planted at about 60 cm from row to row and 30 cm within the row. About 40 to 50 thousand cuttings are required to plant one hectare. In northern India, the cuttings are planted during June-July and in central and southern India during October-November. In some parts, both kharif and rabi crops are grown. A mixture of about 60 kg each of nitrogen and phosphorus and 120 kg of potash per hectare may be applied to obtain good yield. Both flat beds and ridges are used in various parts from 10 to 15 thousand kg per hectare. Red-skinned roots generally store better than white-skinned ones.

The commonest diseases is stem-rot which is spread through soil or diseased roots or vines. The best method of conteolling the diseases is to use diseases-free planting material, and resistant varieties and follow a long crop rotation. Sweet-potato weevil and leaf-eating caterpillars are the most damaging insect pests. The control measures consist in planting roots and cuttings free from weevils and dipping the cuttings before planting into a DDT solution or a mixture of 500 g of lead arsenate in 50 liters of water and spraying the crop with lead arsenate at fortnightly intervals.

Okra or Bhindi

The okra(Abelmoschus esculentus (L.) Moench), belongs to the family Malvaceae. It is cultivated throughout India for its immature fruits. Its varieties are: 'Pusa Sawani', 'Pusa Makhmali', 'Perkin's Long Green' (for hills only), etc.

Cultivation

Bhindi plant prefers a long warm season. The plant is tender and cannot tolerate cold at any stage of growth. Low temperature true in the early spring results in poor germination of seed. Bhindi seed does not germinate at 20^{0}C or below. The best germination takes place between 24^{0}C nad 30^{0}C.

Soil and Soil Preparation

Bhindi can be grown on all kinds of soil except light sandy soil. Well-drained loamy soil rich in organic matter is, however, preferred. Presence of sufficient amount of organic matter improves the nutrient status, soil structure and water holding capacity. Operations for the preparations of land for bhindi sowing would depend upon the condition of the plot. If the plot was under crop which left behind stubbles and the organic material, it has to be ploughed or disced before cultivator is used. In such land normally the disc should be used twice and the tiller three or four times. Two to three plankings would give the desirable structure of the soil. However, if the land was under a crop as potato, one disc operation followed by 3-4 times cultivation would produce the desirable condition of the soil. However, the land has to be planked at least twice before the final sowing is taken up. Sowing is done by two methods:

1. Sowing on ridge
2. Flat sowing.

Sowing on Ridges

This method is particularly important for the early crop sown in february. the field is divided into plots and within each ridges are made 45 cm apart. If possible these should be made running East-West. Seeds are dibbled 1 cm below the soil surface keeping a distance of 15 cm between hills. seed is dibbled on the top of the ridge or slightly on the side facing the sun. This is very important for early crop, as the side facing the sun attains a temperature several degrees haigher than that on the other side. This high temperature affects the seed germination favourably. Ridge sowing for early crop has another advantage. Seeds take many days to germinate and often an irrigation is required to keep up the right moisture content in the soil. In this case pre-emergence irrigation does not lead to crust formation as water is not allowed to run over the ridges.

Flat Sowing

This method is used for the later crop when the days are quite warm. Sowing is done in rows 45 cm apart, which have been previously drilled with fertilizers. Single row cotton drill can also be used efficiently for flat sowing.

This method is quite popular with bhindi seed growers. The advantage of this method over ridge sowing is that it is less labour consuming. Bhindi seed has a hard seed coat. In order to get good germination it is always advisable to soak the seed overnight before sowing. For early crop the soaked seeds may be kept covered at some warm place for sometime so that germination initiates there and slightly sprouted seeds can then be planted in the field.

ESSENTIAL OIL USE IN AROMATHERAPY

Aromatherapy is a form of alternative medicine, in which healing effects are ascribed to the aromatic compounds in essential oils and other plant extracts. Many common essential oils have medicinal properties that have been applied in folk medicine since ancient times and are still widely used today. For example, many essential oils have antiseptic properties, though some are stronger than others.. In addition, many are claimed to have an uplifting effect on the mind, though different essential oils have different properties. The claims are supported in some studies and unconfirmed in others.

Dilution: Essential oils are usually lipophilic (literally: "oil-loving") compounds that usually are not miscible with water. Instead, they can be diluted in solvents like pure 100% ethanol (alcohol), polyethylene glycol, or oils.

Raw Materials: Essential oils are derived from various parts of plants. Some, like orange oil, are derived from any of several parts of the plant.

Berries

- Allspice
- Juniper

Seeds

- Almond
- Anise
- Celery
- Cumin
- Nutmeg oil

Bark

- Cassia
- Cinnamon
- Sassafras

Wood

- Camphor
- Cedar

- Rosewood
- Sandalwood

Rhizome

- Ginger

Leaves

- Basil
- Bay leaf
- Cinnamon
- Common sage
- Eucalyptus
- Lemon grass
- Melaleuca
- Oregano
- Patchouli
- Peppermint
- Pine
- Rosemary
- Spearmint
- Tea tree
- Thyme
- Wintergreen

Resin

- Frankincense
- Myrrh

Flowers

- Chamomile
- Clary sage
- Clove
- Geranium
- Hyssop
- Jasmine
- Lavender
- Manuka
- Marjoram
- Orange
- Rose
- Ylang-ylang

Peel

- Bergamot

- Grapefruit
- Lemon
- Lime
- Orange
- Tangerine

Root

- Valerian

Rose Oil: The most well-known essential oil is probably rose oil, produced from the petals of Rosa damascena and Rosa centifolia. Steam-distilled rose oil is known as "rose otto" while the solvent extracted product is known as "rose absolute".

Dangers: Because of their concentrated nature, EO's generally should not be applied directly to the skin in their undiluted or "neat" form. Some can cause severe irritation or provoke an allergic reaction. Instead, essential oils should be blended with a vegetable carrier oil (also referred to as a base or "fixed" oil) before being applied.

Common carrier oils include olive, almond, hazelnut and grapeseed. Common ratio of essential oil disbursed in a carrier oil is 0.5-3% (most less than 10%) and depends on its purpose. Some EO's including many of the citrus peel oils, are photosensitizers, increasing the skin's reaction to sunlight and making it more likely to burn.

Industrial users of essential oils should consult the material safety data sheets (MSDS) to determine the hazards and handling requirements of particular oils.

Pesticide Residues

There is some concern about pesticide residues in EO's, particularly those used therapeutically. For this reason, many practitioners of aromatherapy choose to buy organically produced oils.

Ingestion: While some advocate the ingestion of essential oils for therapeutic purposes, this should never be done except under the supervision of a professional who is licensed to prescribe such treatment. Some very common EO's such as Eucalyptus are extremely toxic internally. Pharmacopoeia standards for medicinal oils should be heeded. EO's should always be kept out of the reach of children. Some oils can be toxic to some domestic animals, cats in particular. Owners must ensure that their pets do not come into contact with potentially harmful essential oils.

Smoke : The smoke from burning essential oils may contain potential carcinogens, such as polycyclic aromatic hydrocarbons (PAHs). Essential oils are naturally high in volatile organic compounds (VOCs). The internal use of essential oils should be fully avoided during pregnancy without consulting with a licensed professional, as some can be abortifacients in dose 0.5-10 ml.

Media: In 2006, the German movie Perfume: The Story of a Murderer was made on the subject of essential oils. The story takes place in France in the 1700's.

EXTRACTION (FRAGRANCE)

Fragrance extraction refers to the extraction of aromatic compounds from raw materials, using methods such as distillation, solvent extraction, expression, or enfleurage. The results of the extracts are either essential oils, absolutes, concretes, or butters, depending on the amount of waxes in the extracted product.

To a certain extent, all of these techniques tend to distort the odour of the aromatic compounds obtained from the raw materials. Heat, chemical solvents, or exposure to oxygen in the extraction process denature the aromatic compounds, either changing their odour character or rendering them odourless.

Maceration/Solvent Extraction

Certain plant materials contain too little volatile oil to undergo expression, or their chemical components are too delicate and easily denatured by the high heat used in steam distillation. Instead, the oils are extracted using their solvent properties.

Organic Solvent Extraction

Organic solvent extraction is the most common and most economically important technique for extracting aromatics in the modern perfume industry. Raw materials are submerged and agitated in a solvent that can dissolve the desired aromatic compounds. Commonly used solvents for maceration/solvent extraction include hexane, and dimethyl ether.

In organic solvent extraction, aromatic compounds as well as other hydrophobic soluble substances such as wax and pigments are also obtained. The extract is subjected to vacuum processing, which removes the solvent for re-use. The process can lasts anywhere from hours to months. Fragrant compounds for woody and fibrous plant materials are often obtained in this matter as are all aromatics from animal sources.

The technique can also be used to extract odorants that are too volatile for distillation or easily denatured by heat. The remaining waxy mass is known as a concrete, which is mixture of essential oil, waxes, resins, and other lipophilic (oil soluble) plant material, since these solvents effectively remove all hydrophobic compounds in the raw material. The solvent is then removed by a lower temperature distillation process and reclaimed for re-use.

Although highly fragrant, concretes are too viscous - even solid—at room temperature to be useful. This is due to the presence of high-molecular-weight, non-fragrant waxes and resins. Another solvent, often ethyl alcohol, which only dissolves the fragrant low-molecular weight compounds, must be used to extract the fragrant oil from the concrete. The alcohol is removed by a second distillation, leaving behind the absolute. These types of essential oils, from plants such as jasmine and rose, are called absolutes.

Due to the low temperatures in this process, the absolute may be more faithful to the original scent of the raw material, which is subjected to high heat during the distillation process.

Supercritical Fluid Extraction

Supercritical fluid extraction is a relatively new technique for extracting fragrant compounds from a raw material, which often employs Supercritical CO_2 as the extraction solvent. When carbon dioxide is put under high pressure at slightly above room temperature, a supercritical fluid forms (Under normal pressure CO_2 changes directly from a solid to a gas in a process known as sublimation.) Since CO_2 in a non-polar compound has low surface tension and wets easily, it can be used to extract the typically hydrophobic aromatics from the plant material. This process is identical to one of the techniques for making decaffeinated coffee.

Due to the low heat of process and the relatively unreactive solvent used in the extraction, the fragrant compounds derived often closely resemble the original odour of the raw material. Like solvent extraction, the CO_2 extraction takes place at a low temperature, extracts a wide range of compounds, and leaves the aromatics unaltered by heat, rendering an essence more faithful to the original. Since CO_2 is gas at normal atmospheric pressure, it also leaves no trace of itself in the final product, thus allowing one to get the absolute directly without having to deal with a concrete. It is a low-temperature process, and the solvents are easily removed.

In supercritical fluid extraction, high pressure carbon dioxide gas (up to 100 atm.) is used as a solvent.

Ethanol Extraction

Ethanol extraction is a type of solvent extraction used to extract fragrant compounds directly from dry raw materials, as well as the impure oils or concrete resulting from organic solvent extraction, expression, or enfluerage. Ethanol extracts from dry materials are called tinctures, while ethanol washes for purifying oils and concretes are called absolutes.

The impure substances or oils are mixed with ethanol, which is less hydrophobic [than the solutes?] and dissolves more of the oxydized aromatic constituents (alcohols, aldehydess, etc.), leaving behind the wax, fats, and other generally hydrophobic substances. The alcohol is evaporated under low-pressure, leaving behind absolute. The absolute may be further processed to remove any impurities that are still present from the solvent extraction.

Ethanol extraction is not used to extract fragrance from fresh plant materials; these contain large quantities of water, which would also be extracted into the ethanol.

Distillation: Distillation is a common technique for obtaining aromatic compounds from plants, such as orange blossoms and roses. The raw material is heated and the fragrant compounds are re-collected through condensation of the distilled vapour

Today, most common essential oils, such as lavender, peppermint, and eucalyptus, are distilled. Raw plant material, consisting of the flowers, leaves, wood, bark, roots, seeds, or peel, is put into an alembic (distillation apparatus) over water,

Steam Distillation: Steam from boiling water is passed through the raw material for 60-105 minutes, which drives out most of their volatile fragrant compounds. The condensate from distillation, which contain both water and the aromatics, is settled in a Florentine flask.

This allows for the easy separation of the fragrant oils from the water. The water collected from the condensate, which retains some of the fragrant compounds and oils from the raw material. This fragrant water is called hydrosol and is sometimes sold for consumer and commercial use. This method is most commonly used for fresh plant materials such as flowers, leaves, and stems. Popular hydrosols are rose water, lavender water, and orange blossom water. Many plant hydrosols have unpleasant smells and are therefore not sold.

Most oils are distilled in a single process. One exception is Ylang-ylang (Cananga odorata), which takes 22 hours to complete distillation. It is fractionally distilled, producing several grades (Ylang-Ylang "extra", I, II, III and "complete," in which the distillation is run from start to finish with no interruption).

Dry/destructive Distillation: The raw materials are directly heated in a still without a carrier solvent such as water. Fragrant compounds that are released from the raw material by the high heat often undergo anhydrous pyrolysis, which results in the formation of different fragrant compounds, and thus different fragrant notes. This method is used to obtain fragrant compounds from fossil amber and fragrant woods where an intentional "burned" or "toasted" odour is desired.

Expression

Expression as a method of frangrance extraction where raw materials are pressed, squeezed or compressed and the oils are collected. In contemporary times, the only fragrant oils obtained using this method are the peels of fruits in the citrus family. This is due to the large quantity of oil is present in the peels of these fruits as to make this extraction method economically feasible. Citrus peel oils are expressed mechanically, or cold-pressed. Due to the large quantities of oil in citrus peel and the relatively low cost to grow and harvest the raw materials, citrus-fruit oils are cheaper than most other essential oils. Lemon or sweet orange oils that are obtained as by-products of the commercial citrus industry are among the cheapest citrus oils.

Expression was mainly used prior to the discovery of distillation, and this is still the case in cultures such as Egypt. Traditional Egyptian practice involves pressing the plant material, then burying it in unglazed ceramic vessels in the desert for a period of months to drive out water. The water has a smaller molecular size, so it diffuses through the ceramic vessels, while the larger essential oils do not. The lotus oil in Tutankhamen's tomb, which retained its scent after 3000 years sealed in alabaster vessels, was pressed in this manner.

Enfleurage

Enfleurage is a two-step process during which the odour of aromatic materials is absorbed into wax or fat, then extracted with alcohol. Extraction by enfleurage was commonly used when distillation was not possible because some fragrant compounds denature through high heat. This technique is not commonly used in modern industry, due to both its prohibitive cost and the existence of more efficient and effective extraction methods.

CARROT SEED OIL

Carrot seed oil is the essential oil extract of the seed from the carrot plant. The oil is steam distilled from the dried fruit. The odour is a dry-woody, earthy sweet smell, a yellow or amber-coloured to pale orange-brown liquid. Carrot seed oil can be found in different formulas dealing with skin conditions. The oil assists in removing toxins and water build up, giving the skin a fresher tone.

In Aromatherapy

The light yellow to amber coloured essential oil distilled from the seeds (mostly in France, Egypt, and India) differs from the orange carrot oil produced from the root of the common edible carrot. Carrot seed oil nonetheless offers the same familiar scent. Diuretic and hepatic, carrot seed operates as a kidney and liver cleanser, particularly indicated for jaundice and hepatitis. Its depurative (detoxifying) properties are likewise effective for treating arthritis and rheumatism. As a diuretic remedy for genito-urinary ailments, carrot seed is indicated for gout, cystitis, and calculi as well as edema.

Carrot seed stimulates lymphatic circulation and is otherwise carminative and vermifuge, and an emmenagogic menstrual regulator. Its relaxing qualities are helpful in the treatment of premenstual tension. It is also considered a blood tonic indicated for anemia.

As a dermal agent, carrot seed lends its depurative qualities to skin and body care preparations and procedures. A natural tanning agent and skin toner that protects aged and wrinkled skin, carrot seed is also remedial for dermatitis, eczema, psoriasis, and various rashes. It can be used topically to treat boils, abscesses, and skin ulcers.

ANETHOLE

Anethole (or trans-anethole) is an aromatic compound that accounts for the distinctive "licorice" flavor of anise, fennel, and star anise. It may also be referred to as p-propenylanisole, anise camphor, isoestragole, or oil of aniseed. It is unrelated to glycyrrhizic acid, the compound which makes licorice taste sweet. The full chemical name is trans-1-methoxy-4-(prop-1-enyl)benzene. The chemical structure is shown at right. Chemically, it is an aromatic, unsaturated ether.

Anethole appears as white crystals at room temperature. Its melting point is 21 °C, and its boiling point is 234 °C. It has a chemical formula of C10H12O, and is closely related to estragole, an aromatic compound found in tarragon and basil. Anethole is distinctly sweet as well as having its flavoring properties and is measured to be 13 times sweeter than sugar. It is perceived as being pleasant to the taste even at higher concentrations.

It is slightly toxic and may act as an irritant in large quantities. It can stimulate hepatic regeneration in rats, and can also produce spasmolytic activity in high doses. It is a chemical precursor for paramethoxyamphetamine (PMA), which has been sold as ecstasy resulting in several deaths.

EUCALYPTOL

Eucalyptol is a natural organic compound which is a colourless liquid. It is a cyclic ether and a monoterpene. Eucalyptol is also known by a variety of synonyms: 1,8-cineol, limonene oxide, cajeputol, 1,8-epoxy-p-menthane, 1,8-oxido-p-menthane, eucalyptol, eucalyptole, 1,3,3-trimethyl-2-oxabicyclo[2,2,2]octane, cineol, cineole.

Composition: Eucalyptol comprises up to 90 percent of the essential oil of some species of eucalyptus (*e.g.* Eucalyptus polybractea), hence the common name of the compound. It is also found in bay leaves, mugwort, sweet basil, wormwood, rosemary, sage and other aromatic plant foliage. Eucalyptol with a purity from 99.6 to 99.8 percent can be obtained in large quantities by fractional distillation of eucalyptus oil.

Health Warning: In common with all volatile oils (essential oils), eucalyptus oil is toxic if ingested internally.

Properties: Eucalyptol has a fresh camphor-like smell and a spicy, cooling taste. It is insoluble in water, but miscible with ether, ethanol and chloroform. The boiling point is 176 °C and the flash point is 49 °C.

Uses: Because of its pleasant spicy aroma and taste, eucalyptol is used in flavourings, fragrances, and cosmetics. It is also an ingredient in many brands of mouthwash and cough suppressant.

Eucalyptol has been demonstrated to be capable of reducing inflammation and pain. It has also been found to be able to kill leukaemic cells.

Cineol was shown to be an effective treatment for Non-purulent sinusitis in a placebo controlled trial. Laryngoscope. 2004 Apr;114(4):738-42. PMID: 15064633 [PubMed - indexed for MEDLINE] 76 patients per treatment group were assigned to cineole or placebo.

The dosage of the active ingredient was two 100-mg capsules of cineole three times daily. Symptom scores were significantly reduced in the cineole group. The mean values for the symptoms-sum-scores in the cineole group were 6.9 +/- 2.9 after 4 days and 3.0 +/- 2.8 after 7 days, and in the placebo group, 12.2 +/- 2.5 after 4 days and 9.2 +/- 3.0 after 7 days. Treated subjects experienced less headache on bending, frontal headache, sensitivity of pressure points of trigeminal nerve, impairment of general condition, nasal obstruction, and rhinological secretion. Side effects from treatment were minimal.

In a 1994 report released by five top cigarette companies, eucalyptol was listed as one of the 599 additives to cigarettes. It is added to improve the flavor.

AROMATHERAPY

Aromatherapy is the ancient science of healing, relaxing and energizing by the use of plants and their parts. The roots, barks, flowers, fruits, seeds and nuts play a crucial part in this science. It is one of the more popular branches of alternative medicines. The word aromatherapy is derived from two words aroma which means smell and therapy which stands for healing.

Essential oils form the basis of aromatherapy. These essentials oils are the extracts of plants and their parts and form their life force. These oils are extracted by the means of steam distillation, cold expression, or fixed oil or alcohol extraction. They are highly concentrated and should not be used directly. These oils can be blended together and this blend is called synergy. The synergy is more potent than the individual oils combined. To reduce the potency of these oils, you can dilute them by mixing them with carrier oils.

These oils affect your mood. They enter through our olfactory system and affect the nervous system, thus improving mood and relaxing or energizing us. This helps is alleviating stress and speeding up healing. These essential oils also have cosmetic properties and can be used in skincare and hair care products. Many of these oils have known anti-viral, antifungal and antiseptic properties. They are also used in household products for cleaning and antiseptic uses. These oils can be inhaled, massaged onto your body, added to the bath or shower or sprayed in the room.

The essential oils used in aromatherapy are the life force of the plants from which they have been extracted. These oils can be massaged on your body, inhaled, added to your bath or sprayed in the air. When you take "Aromatherapy massage" with the essential oils, these oils are absorbed into the bloodstream via the skin.

Aromatherapy Essential Oils

Aromatherapy oils are popularly known as essential oils. You can use these oils for health, beauty, relaxation and cooking. You can mix two or more essential oils together to form a synergy, while mixing two or more oils together to the vegetable oil can give you blend. You can get the water left after extraction of the oil called hydrosol and use it for healing and beauty purpose. Do not use essential oils directly. Always dilute them with the carrier oils before application. Use only the minimum recommended drops. These oils can be used for cooking and baking, in lieu of vegetable oils and also to add essence to your food. But you need to be careful since these oils are highly volatile. Always keep these oils away from the heat and electric sources as they are highly inflammable. Do not let the children and the pets touch these oils.

What are Essential Oils?

Aromatherapy oils are known as essential oils. These oils are the concentrated extracts of plants and their roots, stems, flowers and fruits. These oils form the base of aromatherapy and influence your body, mind and spirit. Any fragrance that uses an animal product like musk is not pure aromatherapy oil. Similarly, fragrances and perfumes too do not categorize as essential oils though they may smell similar to the aromatherapy oils and do not carry the therapeutic value.

Aromatherapy oils or essential oils are extracted from the plants usually by the means of distillation. The plant matter is treated with steam to soften the plant, break down its tissues and release the pure essential oils. The steam is then cooled down since it contains the essential oils and the water is separated from the oil. This oil is then filtered to get pure aromatherapy oil.

Sometimes they can also be extracted by pressing the part of the plant. *E.g.* if you twist the rind of a lemon or orange, you get a smelly liquid which is the essential oil of the fruit and can be extracted by the presses. The price of aromatherapy oils varies greatly, depending on the number of plant parts used in manufacture.

The greater the number of part plants used higher is the price. Also the oils extracted from the exotic plants are expensive. Lemon oil is cheaper since the rind of lemon contains a lot of oil. But the lavender oil is expensive because flowers contain very little oil and it takes about 45 kilograms of lavender flowers to extract a pound of lavender essential oil. Jasmine, rose and lavender are the most expensive of aromatherapy oils.

Only a few pure essential oils like lavender and tea tree can be applied directly to the skin. The rest of the oils are concentrated and must be diluted by mixing up with carrier oils which are made from nuts and seeds like apricot kernel, grape seed and jojoba, before application.

You can benefit from the use of aromatherapy oils in wide variety of ways like inhaling the oil, massaging it on your body and by soaking yourself in the bath water to which are added the essential oils. Massaging the oil onto the body is the most common method of getting the benefit of aromatherapy oils, since skin is the largest absorption organ that you have.

Oil Profiles

Aromatherapy makes use of different types of essential oils for curing different problems. Essential oils are extracted natural plants and herbs found the in nature. Discovered in the year 1930 by a French scientist it heals people using the aromas of different plants and herbs.

Since essential oils are natural and herbal they are completely safe and do not have any negative side effects.

Angelica Root: Its botanical name is Angelica archangelica. It is extracted by steam distillation. Its colour is pale yellow and it's a thin liquid. It is mainly use for dull skin, exhaustion, gout, toxin buildup, water retention etc. It is phototoxic therefore should be avoided during pregnancy and diabetes.

Anise: Its Botanical Name is Pimpinella anisum. It is extracted by steam Distillation. Its colour is clear and it is a thin liquid. It is used for Bronchitis, colds, coughs, flatulence, flu, muscle aches, rheumatism. Those who have hypersensitive skin should avoid using it. It should also be avoided in endometriosis and estrogen-dependent cancers. It is narcotic and slows circulation if taken in large doses.

Basil: Its botanical name is Ocimum basilicum. It is extracted by steam Distillation. Its colour is clear and it is a thin liquid. It can be used for Bronchitis, colds, coughs, exhaustion, flatulence, flu, gout, insect bites, insect repellent, muscle aches, rheumatism, and sinusitis. High doses of basil may be carcinogenic due to its methyl chavicol content. It should be avoided during pregnancy and liver problems.

Cedarwood Atlas: Its botanical name is cedrus atlantica. It is extracted by steam Distillation. It is light golden yellow in colour and a medium oily liquid. It could be used for Acne, arthritis, bronchitis, coughing, cystitis, dandruff, dermatitis, stress. It should be avoided during pregnancy.

Eucalyptus: Its botanical name is eucalyptus globules. It is extracted by steam Distillation. Its colour is clear and it is a thin liquid. It could be used for Arthritis, bronchitis, catarhh, cold sores, colds, coughing, fever, flu, poor circulation, and sinusitis. It is very toxic when taken orally.

USES FOR ESSENTIAL OILS

Essential oils are the oils extracted from the natural plants and herbs. Aroma of these essential oils is used for aromatherapy. Discovered in the year 1930 by French scientist, aromatherapy is a very good natural technique for rejuvenating human mind and body. The aroma of essential oils directly affects the mental and physical health of the patient. Essential oils also help in creating emotional balance in emotionally disturbed people. These essential oils are highly volatile therefore one need to take great care for storing them.

Some of the essential oils are:

Eucalyptus, Sandalwood, Cedarwood, etc. All essential oils have different characteristics and hence are used for curing different types of disease. Essential oils could be used for curing physical and mental problems of people. It could be used for perfumes, room sprays, toners, shampoos, soaps etc. On the emotional front essential oils such as bergamot, chamomile, juniper, lemon, could be used for easing aggression. Oils such as Jasmine and Rose can be used to ease jealously. Essential oils such as marjoram and Benzoin are helpful for relaxing a person suffering loneliness. Essential oils such as cedarwood, ginger and fennel are effective in treating fear. Essential oils are effective in easing many other unpleasant emotions.

Essential oils can also be used for skin care and treating asthma, warts etc. Apart from curing and healing diseases, essential oils could be used for many other purposes. At home essential could also be used to fragrance wardrobe, book shelves.

It could also be used for preparing insect repellent. Add about 20 drops of essential oils to carrier oil like almond for massaging the body. To keep bookworms away from the books keep patchouli oil near the old books. Spicy oils added to a kettle or simmering water could be used to humidify and freshen the house.

How to Use Essential Oils

You can use aromatherapy essential oils at home or work place in a number of ways. Some of the common ways are:

Aroma therapy Inhalation - Is a process where you add 2-3 drops of essential oil into boiling water and inhale the steam, by covering your head with a towel to stop the steam from escaping. This also opens the pores of the skin and so more oil is absorbed giving the benefits of a facial.

You can place the same bowl containing hot water and aroma oil under your bed so that your entire room is surrounded with aromatic fragrance. Handkerchiefs sprinkled with a drop or two of aroma oil is also beneficial. Similarly a tissue with aromatic oil can also be kept inside a pillow or cushion to have a relaxed and peaceful sleep.

Diffusers or Vaporizers: Diffusers are usually made of clay. They have an opening where you can place candles or earthen lamps. The top portion is like a cup useful for holding water and a few drops of aromatic oil.

Fill in the cup with water, few drops of aromatic oil. Then light candle or lamp filled with castor oil so that it burns for a longer time. The whole atmosphere is filled with fragrance once the water and oil heat up and evaporation takes place for nearly 6 hours. This can be used wherever scented air is required like gatherings, hotels, living rooms and even bedrooms. When the right essential oil is used there is an instant relief from pain and a relaxed positive feeling prevails.

Vaporizers are the insect repellents normally used in the forms of mats can be reused by the addition of 2-3 drops of essential oil and lighting them electrically. Slowly the soothing aroma is dispersed in the entire room. Citronella is used for repelling the insects lavender for bedroom, lemon or rosemary are useful for offices. Tea-tree due to its antiseptic property can be used to disinfect a sick room.

Massage : Aromatherapy Massage gives us the simultaneous double benefits of touch therapy with scent therapy. Massage tones the muscles, releases energy from tense muscles, detoxifies toxins and above all, improves blood circulation. There is a sense of pleasure and well being when you inhale the fragrance. During massage a high amount of oil is able to penetrate through the skin. Usually aroma oils are mixed with carrier oils like olive oil, sweet almond, sesame, coconut, sunflower and vegetable oil. Aroma oils should be used only after dilution, 10 drops or 1 tsp of essential oil can be mixed with 30ml of carrier oil for a rejuvenating effect.

Baths: You can add only a few drops of the selected aromatherapy bath oil to your bathtub or bucket. Stir well since some of the aroma oils are insoluble in water and spend 20 minutes in the tub. The aroma oil enters the body through the skin and gives a relaxed lasting effect.

Foot Bath: After a hard days work you can have a very refreshing feeling by dipping your feet in a bowl of lukewarm water with 2-3 drops of essential oil. This is useful even for sweaty and smelly feet.

Pot Pourri : This is a combination of dried flowers, herbs grass and seed pods to which a few drops of essential oil is added and kept in a bowl to give aromatic fragrance for 4-6 weeks. Another method is to keep the pot pourri mixture along with the essential oil in a container overnight and open the box the next morning so that the aroma spreads in the entire area.

Bed Time : 2-3 drops on the pillow cover while sleeping, is useful in treating headaches, stress, tension and in boosting confidence.

Essential and Organic Oils

Amrette Seed: These have warmth- giving, relaxing and stimulating properties. 2-3 drops of oil are used to relieve anxiety, depression, tiredness and other stress related conditions, cramps, pains and muscular aches. Can freshen up tired and hurting feet. Should be used in low dosage and frequent massages and bath with it should be avoided.

Aniseed: Have warming and stimulating properties. 3-5 drops are helpful in treating bronchitis, coughs and catarrh.

Angelica: Angelica is useful in muscular pains and aches, rheumatism, flu, cold, cough and aides digestion. Used in healing smoker's cough. Not to be used during pregnancy and avoid exposure to sunlight.

Basil: Have uplifting and refreshing properties. Has multiple uses 2-3 drops help to relieve tension, stress, mild anxiety, loss of appetite, indigestion, flatulence, nausea, temporarily relieves cough, sinusitis, cold, fever, bronchitis, earaches, eases rheumatic, arthritic, muscular pains and spasm. It also used as an insect repellent. But is to be avoided during pregnancy.

Bergamot: (3-5 drops) Has calming, refreshing and rejuvenating properties. Can heal wounds, relieves ulcers, treats pre menstrual tension and eczema. Acts as an appetizer. Relieves respiratory infections, colic, flatulence and indigestion. Used in oily skin problems. Used in treating mental and psychological disturbances. It is effective in treating cold sores and chicken pox. Acts as an antiseptic for urinary tract problem. Can be photosensitive and can cause skin irritation.

Black Pepper: Can be warming and strengthening. 2-3 drops can relieve stiffness, pains, muscular aches and fatigue. Helps in curing heartburn, indigestion, flatulence, colic and loss of appetite. Tones muscles and helps in peripheral circulation. Increases concentration and alertness. Provides temporary relief from respiratory infections, chills, cold, flu, arthritis, fibrosis and catarrh. But should used in moderation.

Camphor: Should be used in moderation. Helps in treating colds, coughs, fever, constipation, arthritis, rheumatism, sprains, insomnia, acne, inflamed skin and depression. 2-3 drops can be used at a time.

Cardamom: 2-3 drops can be used. It is a tonic and helps to relieve aches, headaches, coughs, nausea and indigestion. But should be used in moderation.

Chamomile : (3-5) drops can give a soothing effect. Used for diarrhea, gastritis, colitis, urinary tract infection, menopause and menstrual related problems. Eases fear, anxiety and anger. It is helpful in treating sleeplessness and helps to relieve muscular and joint pains and is used in treating skin problems. Soothes inflamed wounds, broken capillaries, blisters. It can be used to lighten fair hair. Has mild effect on children facing teething problem and earache.

Clove Bud: 1-2 drops when used have warming and soothing properties. It is used as an effective antiseptic, analgesic and anti-bacterial. It provides relief from sprains, asthma, cold, flu, dyspepsia, diarrhea, toothache, ulcers, wounds, bronchitis, nervous tension, depression and stress. It is useful in fighting acne and acts as mosquito repellent. It should be used in low moderation and is to be avoided during pregnancy.

Cypress: 2 drops of this can provide refreshed, calm and strengthening effect. It brings down external bleeding, excessive perspiration and heavy menstrual flow; used as an astringent to circulation, hemorrhoids, varicose veins; useful in asthma, bronchitis, dry cough, cold and flu. Helps to heal swollen breasts. It should not be used during pregnancy.

Clarysage : Clarysage has Euphoric, sensual, warming and relaxing properties. 2-5 drops can be used. Brings down high blood pressure and excessive sebum. It is useful in dealing with anxiety, stress, tension and migraine, menstrual cramps and pain, PMT, muscular tension and excessive perspiration. It encourages labour and eases childbirth. Immune system is strengthened and reduces asthma. Causes drowsiness, so it has to be avoided if one suffers from epilepsy or in case of pregnancy.

Eucalyptus: 2-3 drops of this have cooling and clearing properties. It cures cold and fever. Clears blocked nose and head. Relieves stress, fatigue, muscular pains, sprains, aches, rheumatism, headaches, sinusitis and mild respiratory infections. It has anti-inflammatory and antibacterial properties too. And is also used as an insect repellent. Sometimes it can cause skin irritation.

Fennel have calming effect. 2-3 drops are useful in easing colic, constipation, nausea, flatulence, loss of appetite, fluid retention, menstrual pain, PMT, menopause and digestion problems. Has mild laxative and diuretic effect. Cures kidney stones and relieves intestinal spasm. Increases flow of breast milk, relieves bronchitis and helps to fight hangovers. It is to be avoided during pregnancy.

Frankincense it has strengthening and soothing properties. 3-5 drops can be used at a time. Helps in meditation. Strengthens emotionally against grief, fear and nightmares. It cures asthma, bronchitis, coughs and catarrh. It helps in healing dry, wrinkled, scarred, inflamed skin, ulcers and infected wounds. It helps to maintain supple skin.

Geranium : It is associated with calm, balancing, relaxing and refreshing properties. 5-7 drops helps to deal menopausal problems, postnatal depression, PMT. Normalizes skin imbalances and problems. Treats swollen and painful breasts, fluid retention problems, throat infections. It cures cold, flu, acne, bruises, burns, cuts, mouth ulcers, eczema and dermatitis. It acts as astringent and cleanser. Also works as insect repellent.

Ginger: 2-3 drops have warm and stimulating properties. Helps in blood circulation, aids memory, relaxes blood vessels. If inhaled, relieves morning sickness. Relieves pains, aches, sprains and strains. Cures cold, catarrh, flu, fever and sore throat. Relieves flatulence, travel sickness, indigestion. It may cause irritation in sensitive skin so use in moderation.

Juniper Berry: 2-3 drops can be used to heal bruises, acne, colic, cramps, menstrual pain, cough, arthritis, less menstrual flow, swollen and painful breasts. Tones the skin and deals with obesity, loss of appetite, hemorrhoids, poor circulation and fluid retention. If used in excess can irritate kidneys. Not be used if suffering from high B.P. and in pregnancy.

Lavender: It has harmonizing, soothing, balancing, refreshing, relaxing and calming properties. 5-10 drops relieves muscular aches and pains, bites and stings. Cures cold, flu, sleeplessness, headache and minor burns. It helps in relieving anxiety, stress and irritability. It helps to balance and harmonize the body. Usage should be avoided during pregnancy.

Lemon: 3-6 drops help in healing cold, fever, flu, sore throat, mouth ulcers, poor circulation, high B.P., hormonal headaches, wounds, stress, nervous tension, acidity and bronchial problems. Helps to stop hot flushes during menopause. Helps to clear freckles and is an effective insect repellent too. Avoid using it in sunlight.

Lemongrass: (1-3 drops) It helps to open the skin pores, treating oily skin, curing acne and indigestion. Helps in shock, grief and stress. Helps to fight lethargy, insomnia and irritability during menopause, excitability in children. Improves skin elasticity, scars and stretch marks. It gives relief from sore throat, headaches and mild respiratory problems. Can cause skin irritation. To be avoided during pregnancy.

Marjoram: (3-5 drops) Calming to the nervous system. Heals bruises and reduces sexual urges. Relieves anxiety, stress, high B.P., cold, flu, sinusitis, arthritis, rheumatism and swollen joints. Cures indigestion, constipation, flatulence, migraines, stomach and menstrual cramps. Use in limit and avoid during pregnancy.

Neroli: (1-3 drops) Helps in shocks, trauma, grief, stress, menopause and PMT. Cures dryness, improves elasticity of the skin. Calms restless children. Helps to lighten stretch marks and scars. Helps during pregnancy and labour.

Orange (sweet): (2-3 drops) Gentle on children and brings down fever. Eases constipation and diarrhea. Treats nervous tension, stress and anxiety, effective in healing mouth ulcers. Gives relief from bronchial coughs, colds, flu and insomnia. Avoid using under sunlight.

Palmarosa: (4-5 drops) Relieves cold, flu, indigestion, viruses and reduces fever. Helpful in treating acne, scars, dermatitis, maintains supple skin. Stimulates circulation, cell regeneration and appetite.

Tea Tree: (2-5 drops) helpful in treating colds, flu, cold sores, shock, burns, bacterial and viral infections, nappy rash, stings, herpes, hysteria and in healing fungal and yeast infections.

Thyme (White) : (2 drops) A good stimulant and expectorant. Helpful in relieving cold, coughs, tension, anxiety, fatigue, skin irritation, headaches, rheumatic aches and pains. Also an useful insect repellent.

Vetiver: (1-3 drops) Heals cuts, wounds, blemishes and acne. Helpful in relieving stress, sprains, tension, muscular aches, pains, arthritis, rheumatism, stiffness, palpitations and congestion.

Ylang Ylang: (2-3 drops) Useful in skin care, high B.P., insomnia, PMT, menopause, impotence, frigidity, scalp conditioner. Helps to relieve stress, anxiety, tension, uncontrolled anger, rapid breathing and heart rate. If taken in excess it may cause headache and nausea. Not to be used before driving.

Bibliography

Akerele, O.: *Medicinal plants: policies and priorities*, Cambridge, UK; Cambridge University Press, 1991.

Chandrasekar B: *Blood sugar lowering potentiality of selected Cucurbitaceae plants of Indian origin*. Ind J Med Res. 1989.

Chattopadhyay RR: *A comparative evaluation of some blood sugar lowering agents of plant origin*. J Ethnopharmacology. 1999.

De Silva T.: *A Manual on the Essential Oil Industry*, Vienna, Austria; United Nations Industrial Development Organisation, 1996.

Donellan, C.: *Endangered species*. Independence, Cambridge, 1995.

Dutt, Ashwini : *An Introduction to Medicinal Plants*, Adhyayan Pub, Delhi, 2008.

Featherly H. I.: *Taxonomic Terminology of the Higher Plants*, USA, Iowa State College Press, 1954.

Felig G, Bergman M, Felig C.: *The Endocrine Pancreas: Diabetes mellitus*, New York: MacGraw-Hill; 1995.

Fitzsimmons, Judith : *Seasons of Aromatherapy: Hundreds of Restorative Recipes and Sensory Suggestions.* Conari Press, Berkeley, CA; 1998

Fuller, D.: *Medicine from the Wild*. Washington, DC; Traffic USA, 1991.

Godden G.: *Growing Citrus Trees*, Australia, Lothian Publishing Company Pvt. Ltd., 1988.

Goldsmith, F.B.: *Monitoring for conservation and ecology.* Chapman and Hall, London, 1991.

Harlan, Jack R.: *The Living Fields: Our Agricultural Heritage*, Cambridge: Cambridge University Press, 1998.

Hartley W.: *A Checklist of Economic Plants in Australia*, Melbourne, C.S.I.R.O., 1979.

Hessayon D. G. Dr.: *The Vegetable Expert*, England, PBI, Publications, 1985.

Heywood, V. & Synge, H.: *Conservation of medicinal plants*. Cambridge Univ. Press, Cambridge, UK, 1991.

Hill, Clare: *The Ancient and Healing Art of Aromatherapy.* Ulysses Press, Berkeley, CA; 1997.

Janardhanan, K.K. : *Diseases of Major Medicinal Plants*, Daya, Delhi, 2002.

Janick, Jules: *Horticultural Science*, New York: W. H. Freeman and Company, 1986.

Jeet Inder : *Rainwater Harvesting*, Mittal, Delhi, 2009.

Jeffers P.: *Evaluation of Four Onion Varieties in Montserrat*, Plymouth, CARDI, 1992.

Jerram, M.R.K. : *A Text-Book on Forest Management : In Agriculture, Horticulture and Forestry*, Asiatic Pub, Delhi, 2006.

Kalia Manoranjan : *Post Harvest Technology of Vegetables*, Agrotech Pub, Delhi, 2006.

Karnick, C.R. : *Ayurvedic Narcotic Medicinal Plants*, Sri Satguru, Delhi, 1996.

Kim J. S.: *Sources of Resistance to Viruses of Pepper (Capsicum spp.): a Catalogue*, Taipei, AVRDC, 1994.

Kumar, Supriya : *Amenity Horticulture, Biotechnology and Post-Harvest Technology*, Pointer, Delhi, 2006.

Lawless, Julia: *Essential Oils: An Illustrated Guide.* Harpercollins, London, 2001.

Lewington, A.: *Medicinal Plant and Plant Extracts*, Cambridge, UK; Traffic International, 1993.

Mabberley D. J.: *The Plant-Book : a Portable Dictionary of the Vascular Plants*, Cambridge, Cambridge University Press, 1997.

Madulid Domingo A.: *A Pictorial Cyclopedia of Philippine Ornamental Plants*, Philippines, Makati Metro Manila, 1995.

Matsuoka H.: *Cultivation of Panicum Genetic Resources for Evaluation of Characteristics*, Tokyo, JICA, 1997.

McGilvery, Carole and Reed, Jimi: *The Complete Guide to Aromatherapy.* Lorenz Books, London, 2001.

Mellor, J. W.: *The New Economics of Growth*, Ithaca, Cornell University Press, 1976.

Morton Julia F.: *Fruits of Warm Climates*, Miami, Julia F. Morton Publisher, 1987.

Myers, N.: *The Sinking Ark: A New Look at the Problem of Disappearing Species*. Oxford, UK; Pergamon Press, 1979.

Narayan Das Prajapati: *A Handbook of Medicinal Plants*, Agrobios, Delhi, 2005.

Nayar, M.P.: *Hot Spots of Endemic Plants of India, Nepal and Burma.* The Director, TBGRI, Trivandrum, 1996. 252 pp.

Oka H. I.: *Origin of Cultivated Rice*, Elsevier, Japan Scientific Societies Press, 1988.

Oldham P.: *Cost of Production of Major Tree Crops in Dominica*, Roseau, Ministry of Agriculture, 1991.

Panda S.C. : *Post Harvest Technology and Farm Mechanization*, Agrobios, Delhi, 2008.

Percival John: *The Wheat Plant - A Monograph*, London, Duckworth & Co., 1921.

Peter, K.V. : *Basics of Horticulture*, New India, Delhi, 2009.

Pilgrim R.: *Post Harvest Handling of Minor Exotics*, St. George's, Grenada, 1996.

Raffauf R.F.: *The Healing Forest: Medicinal and Toxic Plantsm*, Portland, Oregon, USA; Dioscorides Press, 1990.

Index

❑❑❑